# HARNESS THE POWER OF SELF CARE

## A guide to Regaining Control of your Life.

# Table of Contents

**PART A**

## INTRODUCTION

"Self-care" is a common buzzword these days, but what exactly does it imply? If you look on social media or in a magazine, it may seem that the idea of self-care is nothing more than an excuse to indulge in luxury or to treat yourself in some way. However, there is much more to it than that.

Self-care is the practice of telling yourself what you want – physically, psychologically, or emotionally – and ensuring that you receive it. It is not necessarily selfish or indulgent; it is important. We are solely responsible as adults for our fitness, feelings, and personal development. Self-care is a collection of activities that enables one to do so.

### Why Do You Take Care of Yourself?

"Put on your oxygen mask before helping others," flight attendants advise. This word of warning is an excellent metaphor for self-care. Modern life makes it easy to neglect your well-being to keep up with other commitments, but doing so is unsustainable and even dangerous in the long run.

Perhaps you've witnessed one of the following common symptoms of not taking care of yourself:

Compassion fatigue is a form of exhaustion that impairs the ability to feel joy and sincere concern for others. It is hard to be thankful and truly present for your loved ones when you are physically, mentally, emotionally, or spiritually exhausted. Compassion exhaustion is the equivalent of attempting to pour from an empty cup.

Burnout is a condition of persistent stress caused by overwork. A job often causes burnout, but it may also be caused by school, family life, or other forms of occupation. Physical and mental fatigue, feelings of cynicism, irritability, or rigidity, and various states of "inoperability" – feeling inefficient, disconnected, or useless – are all symptoms. Burnout sometimes results in unhealthy self-medication.

Inadequate physical fitness. Physical self-care includes everything from doctor's appointments to healthy meal preparation and exercise and wellness courses. If you ignore these behaviors, you will inevitably undergo an avoidable decline. Furthermore, a lack of self-care contributes to increased tension, which has physical consequences. Obesity, high blood pressure, heart disease, diabetes, and other conditions are all exacerbated by stress.

The first step toward quality self-care is to understand what it is and why it is essential. So, if you're reading this, I'd like to congratulate you! You've already begun your journey.

The following move is to assume that you are deserving of it, which is easier said than done. We'll say it again: taking care of yourself does not make you greedy, poor, or inferior in any way. Only you can manage your own life. You have to look after yourself. And, as we always say, you deserve to feel better.

Learning to quiet your inner critic – the little voice in your head that says, "It's not worth it," "You should be doing more," or "Everyone else is doing better" – is an important part of this process. These critical, judgmental, and self-blaming phrases reinforce the message that you are insufficient and keep you feeling insignificant and worthless. To confront this voice and know it isn't valid. It's just a hunch. If you make an unhealthy decision now and then, don't beat yourself up about it. Be gentle with yourself, forgive yourself, and make plans for doing better the next time.

If you want to take better care of yourself but don't know where to start, try a self-exploration or reflection exercise to determine where you stand to benefit the most.

## Self-Evaluation Questions

- Do you get enough sleep?

- Are you feeding your body well and drinking plenty of water?

- Do you engage in daily exercise? Do you get enough exercise in your everyday life?

- Are you happy with your relationships? If you have a social support network?

It's tempting to try to do too much self-care at once when you're feeling optimistic. Keep in mind that developing behaviors requires time, effort, and mindfulness. Begin small and check in with yourself regularly.

Create a plan for those S.O.S. moments when you're feeling depressed or frustrated by the various positions you perform, in addition to your regular self-care activities. Consider: what routines and events make you feel at ease? Where do you feel most secure? Who are the people who lift you and encourage you?

Make a list of the things and experiences that make you happy. Consider scenarios in which you are at home, at work, or on the road. Workplace self-care is as essential as personal self-care, particularly if your job is taxing or stressful.

# PART A

## SELF CARE

## YOUR SELF-ESTEEM DETERMINES YOUR LIFE

Perhaps the most vital aspect of the psychology of time management and the role that your self-concept plays in identifying your success and behavior is the effect of your self-esteem in finding out what happens to you. The majority of psychotherapists concur that self-esteem is the crucial determinant of a healthy and balanced individuality. The simplest definition of self-esteem is how much you like yourself." Because you appreciate and value yourself, you still do and behave far better than if you didn't.

The better you like yourself, the more confidence you have. The more you like yourself, the more efficient and reliable you are in each area of your life. Self-esteem is the key to peak performance.

Your self-esteem is so important to your psychological well-being that almost everything you do is meant to increase your feelings of self-esteem and individual worth or to shield it from being reduced by other individuals or scenarios. Self-esteem, the sense of liking, and appreciating yourself are the structural principles of success and joy. It is essential for you to feel active.

## The Trick to Optimal Performance

The flip side of self-esteem is called self-efficiency." It is described as how effective you know you will do or have a task or a job. When you feel that you are proficient at something, you experience favorable feelings of self-efficacy.

Among the best discoveries in psychology was the discovery of the link between self-esteem and also self-efficacy. Currently, we know that the more you like on your own, the much better you do at almost anything you attempt. And too, the better you do at something, the much more you like yourself.

Each eats as well as strengthens the various other. This searching for is what makes time administration so crucial for every component of your life. The better you utilize your time, the more you get done, and also, the higher is your sense of self-efficacy. As a result, you like yourself extra, do even higher quality work, as well as get even a lot more done. Your whole life boosts.

**Three additional elements influence your self-worth that relates to time monitoring.**

- *Determine Your Values*

Living your life consistent with your values is important for you to take pleasure in high self-esteem. Individuals who are clear about what they rely on and worth and decline to endanger their values respect themselves even more than those who are vague regarding what is truly crucial.

It right away raises the concern, "How much do you value your life?" Individuals who value their lives are individuals that extremely value themselves. Individuals that value themselves very utilize their time well. They understand that their time is their life.

The "Legislation of Reversibility" claims that sensations and activities connect on each various other. If you feel a certain means, you will certainly act in a manner consistent you're your feeling. Nonetheless, the reverse is also true.

If you behave in a certain manner, your acts will certainly create the feelings that accompany them inside you. It implies that when you behave as though your time was incredibly important, the action will make you feel like a more valuable and vital person. By handling your time well, you increase your self-confidence, and also, by extension, you progress at whatever you are doing.

The very act of living your life regularly with your worth, as well as using your time successfully and well, improves your self-image, builds your self-esteem and self-confidence, and raises your self-respect.

- *Strive for Proficiency*

The second variable that affects your self-esteem is your feeling of being in control of your life and work; your sense of proficiency in whatever you do.

Whatever you learn more about time management and afterward use in your work triggers you to feel more in control of yourself and your life. As a result, you feel more reliable and also effective. You feel much more productive and also effective. Every increase in your sensation of effectiveness and productivity increases your self-confidence and boosts your sense of individual wellness.

- ### *Know What You Want*

The 3rd aspect that directly influences your self-worth is your current goals and objectives and the tasks you take to achieve those goals. The even more your goals and your activities agree with your worth, the much better you feel. When you are working on something that you believe in, and that is compatible with your all-natural talents and abilities, you like on your own a lot more, and also, you do your work better.

# How self-esteem increases your productivity

Have you, or any person you recognize, effectively handled to grow a cedar tree from a melon seed? The answer is probably no. I'm so specific about this since one legislation of nature is that you reap what you sow. A lot of you are possibly assuming, "Duh. That is evident, right? "My answer is: It cannot be that evident because many individuals are constantly trying to obtain a free ride.

Employees in organizations, supervisors in significant firms, and human beings will constantly want much more and desire it for free if they can get it. Individuals prefer more yet don't intend to place the effort it requires actually to create value.

I'm not also particular that the suggestion of value creation is extensively understood.

## What is value creation?

Value creation isn't simply showing up at eight and also leaving at 5. It relies on what you do during that time. For instance, did you arrive late to work, eat a morning meal, talk to close friends concerning what went down last evening or over your weekend, spend hours surfing the Internet, take several restrooms and also cigarette breaks, remain at lunch longer than you're intended to, and afterward shut down mind and body before the day's end? These tasks are subtracting worth.

Studies verify that the majority of workers are no more than 50 percent efficient at the workplace! It is such a waste of resources and life generally. You invest 35 percent of your life in the office.

## How do you increase your earnings?

To increase your income, you have to be effective for everyone when you're at work. All of your jobs need to be high-value ones, and advancement and success are most likely to follow. A few instances of value-adding tasks are: decreasing the cost of a job, service, or item; discovering an imaginative remedy to an issue; resolving a conflict; creating a new service or product; doing points extra accurately and faster; as well as closing a rewarding sale.

One excellent day-to-day exercise involves documenting five to 10 successes you've attained day by day's end. It assists in recognizing on an exceptionally personal degree what value creation will suggest. Value creation is everything about addition, not a reduction. "You reap what you sow" puts on all facets of your life, which include your task.

## How to turn around reduced self-esteem

Researches have shown that most of the globe's problems might be mapped to a single core cause: low self-worth.

You have viewpoints about, and also an image of, on your own as an individual. This picture or concept consists of the basis of your self-worth and absolutely affects how you feel around, and thus just how much worth you put on yourself. But your self-confidence isn't uncompromising, as well as the way you think can constantly transform.

<u>Looking for the excellent, declaring, or at the very least looking for what might be gained from each experience is a superb beginning factor for improving your self-esteem. Being unfavorable or being positive is a habit.</u>

If you're unfavorable, you're more likely to have lower self-esteem because you focus more on the mistakes you have actually made and also your perceived weaknesses. On the other hand, if you're confident, you're likely to have more trust in yourself since you will certainly watch yourself in a much more favorable means.

If you think about the statement that many problems may be traced to low self-worth, you're able to see it as a practical core to the issues of bad efficiency, low performance, and resistance to change.

## <u>People with high self-esteem are likelier to be successful</u>

Individuals with high self-confidence are more likely to succeed in their individual and professional lives since they add worth. They want to pay the cost-- in initiative, time, and personal financial investment-- of accomplishment to end up being smarter, better, extra well-informed, and more powerful. These individuals' benefits will certainly include individual job and economic incentives, a track record as experts within their services, and acknowledgment for being reliable.

However, the highest possible benefit is going to be completely individual satisfaction in a task well done.

1. How can my self-esteem determine my life?

2. What should be done to increase my earnings?

3. When I turn around, can it reduce my self-esteem?

4. What value does self-esteem add to my productivity?

5. If I have high self-esteem, will I be successful?

**Note yourself Improvement in this chapter**

_____

_____

_____

## MANAGING YOUR STRESS

Are you feeling stressed? You are. You have too much on your plate; due dates are impending, individuals depend on you, and cover it all off, you still have holiday purchasing to do. You are under a great deal of pressure-- so much that sometimes, you suspect the top quality of your job experiences for it.

It is life in the modern work environment. It is impossible to be an expert these days and not experience regular spells of extreme stress and anxiety. The gap between those who excel and those that aren't is not whether you struggle with stress and anxiety but how you deal with it when you do.

Right here are scientifically proven strategies for defeating stress and anxiety whenever it strikes:

# Do i understand what  self-compassion mean?

Self-compassion is, fundamentally, cutting yourself some slack. It's wanting to check out your blunders or failings with compassion and also understanding-- without harsh objection or defensiveness. Research studies reveal that self-compassionate individuals are better, more hopeful, less distressed, and clinically depressed. That's most likely not unusual. However, right here's the twist: they are a lot more effective, also. The majority of us believe that we require to be hard on ourselves to execute at our finest, however it turns out that's 100 percent incorrect. When points are at their most difficult, a dosage of self-compassion can minimize your anxiety and improve your efficiency by making it less complicated to learn from your mistakes. So note that it is human to err and also give yourself a break.

# What do I bear in mind about the "big picture"?

Anything you require or intend to do can be considered in more than one means. As an example, "exercising" can be defined in Broad view terms, like "getting much healthier"-- the why of exercising-- or it can be explained in much more concrete terms, like "running two miles"-- the how of exercising. Believing Broad View regarding the job you do can be very energizing despite anxiety and challenge. You are connecting one certain, often tiny activity to a greater significance or objective. Something that might not appear important or valuable on its own obtains cast in an entirely new light. So when remaining that extra hour at the workplace at the end of a stressful day is thought of as "aiding my profession" instead of "responding to emails for 60 more minutes," you'll be a lot more likely to wish to sit tight as well as work hard.

## Do i rely upon routines?

If I ask you to name the significant root causes of tension in your job life, you would most likely say things like due dates, a heavy workload, bureaucracy, or your awful employer. You possibly wouldn't claim "having to make many choices" because lots of people aren't mindful that this is a powerful and also pervasive root cause of anxiety in their lives. Whenever you choose-- whether it has to do with employing a new worker, about when you create a meeting with your boss, or choosing rye or whole wheat for your egg salad sandwich-- you develop a state of psychological tension actually, stressful. (This is why purchasing is so stressful-- it's not the dreadful concrete floorings, it's all that determining.).

The service is to minimize the number of choices you need to make by using regimens. If there's something you require to do each day, do it at the same time each day. Have a regular plan for your day in the early morning and evacuating to go residence in the evening. Straightforward habits can drastically reduce your experience of anxiety. President Obama that assuredly knows a good deal regarding pressure pointed out using this method himself in an interview:

You require to get rid of from your life the day-to-day issues that soak up many people for significant parts of their day. You'll see I use just grey or blue fits. I'm trying to pare down decisions. I don't intend to make decisions concerning what I'm consuming or wearing because I have way too many other choices to make. You require to focus your decision-making power. You need to routinize yourself. You cannot be undergoing the day distracted by trivia. -Head of State Obama, Vanity Fair.

## Why should I take 5 (or ten) minutes to do something you find fascinating?

If there were something you could include in your auto's engine so that after driving it a hundred miles, you'd end up with even more gas in the tank than you started with, wouldn't you utilize it? Also, if absolutely nothing like that exists for your auto right now, there is something you can do for yourself that will certainly have the same impact, doing something intriguing. It matters not what it is, as long as it fascinates you. Current research shows that passion doesn't just maintain you are going regardless of fatigue; it renews your energy. After that, replenished energy flows right into whatever you do next.

Keep these two extremely crucial points in mind: First, fascinating is not the same thing as positive, fun, or relaxing (though they are not mutually special.) Taking a lunch break may be comforting, and if the food is good, it will probably be positive. Yet unless you are consuming at the hot brand-new molecular gastronomy dining establishment, it possibly will not be fascinating. So it will not renew your power.

Second, intriguing does not have to indicate uncomplicated. The same studies revealed that the rate of interest restored energy revealed that it did so also when the interesting task was a difficult and necessary effort. So you don't have to "unwind" to re-fill your tank.

## What brings adding where and when to my order of tasks?

Will you have a list of a to-do? (if you have a "Job" bar on the side of your schedule, as well as you utilize it, then the response is "yes.") As well as do you locate that a day or a week (or occasionally longer) will frequently pass by without a single thing getting checked off? Demanding, isn't it? You need a method to get the important things done that you layout to do promptly. What you require is if-then preparation (or what psychologists call "application intentions").

This specific type of planning is a truly effective way to help you accomplish any goal. Nearly 200 researches on every little thing from diet and workout to arrangement and time management have revealed that choosing ahead of time when and where you will complete a task can increase or triple your chances of really doing it.

So take the tasks on your order of business, and include a particular when and were per. For example, "Bear in mind to call Sam" becomes "If it is Tuesday after lunch, then I'll call Sam." Since you've produced an if-then plan for calling Bob, your subconscious mind will certainly start scanning the setting, looking for the circumstance in the "if" part of your list. It enables you to seize the critical moment and also make the phone call, even when you are hectic doing various other things. And again, what better method exists to lower your stress and anxiety than going across points off your to-do list?

## Why am I using if-then for positive self-talk?

One more means to battle tension using if-then strategies is to guide them at the experience of stress and anxiety itself, rather than at its causes. Current studies show that the if-then approach can help us manage our psychological actions to circumstances in which we feel stress, unhappiness, exhaustion, self-doubt, or perhaps disgust. Just choose what sort of response you wish to have instead of feeling anxious and make a plan that links your desired feedback to the situations that elevate your blood pressure. For example, "If I see lots of emails in my Inbox, then I will certainly stay calm as well as kicked back," or, "If a deadline is coming close to, then I will keep an awesome head."

## What do I notice in my work in terms of progression, not perfection?

Most of us approach the goals we seek with either attitude: what I call the Be-Good frame of mind, where the emphasis gets on confirming that you have a lot of capacity which you already understand what you're doing, and the Get-Better mindset, where the focus gets on creating your capability and also learning brand-new skills. You can consider the distinction between wishing to show that you are wise versus intending to get smarter.

When you have a Be-Good frame of mind, you expect to be able to do whatever flawlessly right out of eviction, and you continuously (frequently automatically) contrast yourself to other individuals to see how you "size up." You quickly begin to doubt your capacity when things don't go smoothly, which develops anxiety. Ironically, stressing over your ability makes you much more likely to fall short ultimately.

A Get-Better mindset, on the various other hand, leads instead to self-comparison as well as a concern with making progression-- how well are you doing today, compared to just how you did the other day, last month, or in 2015? When you think about what you are performing in terms of learning and boosting, approving that you might make some mistakes in the process, you experience far less stress and anxiety, and you stay inspired despite the problems that may occur.

## Why should I think about the progress that I've already made?

"Of all things that can increase feelings, inspiration, and also perceptions during a workday, the single essential is making development in meaningful work." It is what Teresa Amabile and Steven Kramer describe as the Progress Concept-- the idea is that it's the "little success" that keeps us going, precisely despite stress factors.

Emotionally, it's commonly not whether we've reached our objective, yet the rate at which we are closing the gap between where we are now and where we intend to end up that figures out just how we feel. It can be significantly practical to take a minute and review what you have accomplished so far before turning your interest in the challenges that stay in advance.

## Do I know whether optimism or defensive pessimism helps you?

It's tough for most of us to stay positive when we have got jobs as much as our eyeballs. For others, it isn't simply hard-- it feels wrong. And as it turns out, they are entirely proper-- optimism doesn't help them.

It is stressful sufficient to try to manage as many tasks and objectives as we do. Yet, we add a layer of tension without understanding it when we try to reach them using techniques that don't feel right-- that do not mesh with our very own motivational design. So what's your motivational style, and is "remaining favorable" right for you?

Some individuals consider their work as chances for achievement and accomplishment-- they have what psychologists call a promotion focus. In the language of economics, promo emphasis is all about making the most of gains as well as staying clear of missing out on opportunities. For others, doing a job well has to do with safety, about not losing the placements they've worked so hard to get. This avoidance emphasis emphasizes preventing risk, satisfying responsibilities, as well as doing what you feel you ought to do. It's about lessening losses in economic terms, attempting to hang on to what you've got.

Understanding promotion and avoidance motivation help us understand why individuals can function differently to reach the same goal. Promo inspiration feels like enthusiasm-- the desire to go all out honestly-- and this enthusiasm is continual and improved by a positive outlook. Believing that whatever is most likely to work out wonderful is essential for promotion-focused efficiency. On the other hand, prevention inspiration seems like vigilance-- the requirement to maintain threat at bay--, and it is sustained not by optimism, however by a sort of protective pessimism. In other words, the prevention-minded function best when they think about what might go wrong and what they can sustain that from taking place.

So, do you spend your life seeking accomplishments as well as awards, grabbing the celebrities? Or are you active in meeting your tasks and duties-- being the person every person can count on? Begin by identifying your focus, and afterward, accept either the sunny outlook or the passionate hesitation that will minimize your tension and maintain your execution at your business.

1. Why do I need to manage my stress?

2. How do I deal with my self-compassion?

3. Do I need to rely on my routine?

## 4. Is it a must I check on my work progression?

## Note yourself Improvement in this chapter

---------------------------------------------------

---------------------------------------------------

---------------------------------------------------

---------------------------------------------------

---------------------------------------------------

---------------------------------------------------

---------------------------------------------------

---------------------------------------------------

---------------------------------------------------

---------------------------------------------------

---------------------------------------------------

---------------------------------------------------

---------------------------------------------------

---------------------------------------------------

---------------------------------------------------

---------------------------------------------------

---------------------------------------------------

---------------------------------------------------

---------------------------------------------------

---------------------------------------------------

---------------------------------------------------

---------------------------------------------------

---------------------------------------------------

---------------------------------------------------

## ANXIETY

"Thinking again if you do not think that your physical health affects your anxiety, depression, sadness, and stress. All those emotions trigger chemical reactions that can cause inflammation and a weakened immune system in your body. Learn how to deal with this, sweet friend. There's always going to be dark days."

Let me share my own experience and explain fear in general before we specifically get to social worry. You can truly appreciate the things that I share about social anxieties with you.

During our church service, I go up on stage to meet more than 1,000 people every week. Many times, I've been given at least seven days before the subject that I'm expected to mention for a given weekend service. But sometimes, I'm just given a day or two to get ready. Even more exciting than that, at the start of the service itself, I have been asked, and still am, to replace the assigned person.

If I say to you – and I'm not bragging – you would believe me, it no longer bothers me whether a week or minutes have I been given to prepare? More – you really would believe me if I told you that once I was a nervous wreck, I even talked to a girl I like or had to talk to anybody? Perhaps you wonder, how would it be? Now, my story is here.

I used to be so, so timid. As I said, it's enough for me to sweat blood even with the prospect of having small talk. To me, it's just as risky to hire a completely random stranger for small but rational talk as to approach the same but to yell on his face, "I'm strange! "How strange, huh?

But it was a long time ago. As I wrote previously, I am now nearly every week on a certain Sunday, where I am standing very comfortably over 1000 people. You might ask what happened. Well, unfortunately, I can't do all the credit that my humble self would like for the 180-degree turn. God's hand brought me to situations that shaped my personality and enabled me to overcome my social anxiety.

I was forced to find answers as to why this happened and seek a way to consolidate itself in life's processes by my dad's unexpected – and in my view, premature – death in 2000. So it was that I was going to have a next orientation seminar in the church for a group of individuals

At that time. At that time. I registered and attended this 13-week program, being the religious person my parents raised me to be.

My first social anxiety baptism of fire came at the end of this 13-week program: Dance in public! I know that this is a joy for most people. But since I was socially uncomfortable and very shy who was as skilled at dancing as Manny Pacquiao's song, it was almost a death experience for me!

I was trying to exercise my right to vote for myself, but I had to be humiliated by dancing before people, all my fellow Group members, voted against my wish.

While in a group, I danced naturally like a log; the attention worsened to me – screaming my name. It is exacerbated the nauseous and anxious feelings. Both puke, and I wanted to hide. But I suppose that God (or any deity in which you believe – or the cosmos) was real! I survived could return to my normal, shy, and remote introverted life. I survived. Or I was thinking so.

The forces in that church community thought I would make great materials for leadership for some strange reason. So I decided to adopt the position of heading the next orientation batch following some pressure from the leaders and an unexpected covenant I had to make with God. It would mean that I will also be the last-minute speaker for each of the 13 weekly talks, apart from supervising other volunteers, if the designated speakers do not. What did I get into me?

And just as I was afraid, a few eloquent speakers could not make their speeches, so I had to unite courageously and speak. There is no option. Even if the group was just ten people, it's like the filled staples center or a Quicken Loans Arena for a socially anxious person. So I delivered the talks after I had prepared my last will and will. And there was another funny thing.

I have survived! I survived.

A couple of more conversations with most of my friends as an audience, with people talking slowly became easier, and I became more comfortable talking to everyone in the process. But I was not as bad as before, and I was still timid and anxious. It was probably because I felt I was talking to as many people that I was ever going to do in my life. I was mistaken, boy.

I moved into another church after several years in that community. As leaders in that church personally knew me, they were all right that I paused the ministry and was a member of it only. But I was eventually asked to speak before the general membership, like the previous one, although this time almost weekly, with a large, less well-known crowd.


Here we're back... mode of anxiety!

The management let me take baby steps was one of the best things that happened at that time. From the rest to the speech tasks once a week. To the weekly one. They finally added the ante and let me preach on certain services from the weekly introduction. I became more and more confident and less anxious – again, not for my efforts but for the people around me who pushed me into the limelight, however softly.


However, it's still not the end. It was at most an 80-man group of people. And since it was a small community church, eventually they became a family, and it became so much like the first time – mostly family and friends, albeit on a larger scale. And I moved to my wife's church when I was married – and that was much larger than mine.

Because it was a big church (we talked about at least 10,000 members who attended eight various weekend celebrations), I felt that I was an ordinary member at home. I was thinking, finally! I mean, I don't think I need to step up and talk on stage, with all the veterans and more eloquent speakers out there. At least not where 1200 people are attending each service on average.

Again, I've been mistaken.

For over two years, I have been led to various groups and leaders, and I have ended up preaching in the group of one of 3 of the 8 Senior Pastors. He did not have people to help him, especially during his preaching transitions and exhortations. Review what? What? I was again assigned to speak, but I was supposed to have passed through the roof with anxiety this time.

Me, are 1,200 people talking? I'm not careful how brief my talks are going to be - 1,200 people! If I was so anxious about ten people on average, I should have been 80 by 15! If I were so anxious about the average crowd!

Can you imagine my level of anxiety in my first ever concert in my present church when I got on stage? I'd probably have if I could sweat blood. Even after I had a whole bottle of water minutes before I flashed, my mouth and throat dry. In my mind, my anxiety seemed flushed away from all my preparations. But there was something else.

The anxiety was not so severe this time. In fact, unlike my first talk before ten people, I did not tank my first 1,200- person on stage. However, I was still distressed and could not do as well as my previous conversations in smaller locations. However, this was a crowd that's fifteen times more comprehensible. The remainder, however, was history. After almost two years, I'm not worried about talking to a crowd or talk to a stranger any further. My social anxiety seems to have gone well. Indeed, I would say that I don't panic or worry about speaking to more than 10,000. It would seem that 1,000 people were the tip of my social anxiety.

## What Is Anxiety?

Simply put, it's an uncertain result, worried, nervous, or uneasy. It is what you felt when you first asked your crush for your first day or when you asked your crush for your very first day or day. It's the same feeling when you first cycle without the training wheels or when your first skydive. You're the very bold type. For those like me, on your wedding day, it's the same feeling, at least your first. Why does this happen? Marriage is no longer the "safe" decision these days, as it used to be, increasing divorce rates worldwide.

However, anxiety is not the same as a catastrophe. In its simplest form, anxiety is only anxiety or nervousness. It is everything there is to it. It is everything. As such, please forgive the pun, but there should be no cause for concern. It's human to be nervous and worried about things like speaking in front of 10,000 or dancing on national television that would usually make most people like this.

However, anxiety disorders are a whole new story.

## Disorders of Anxiety

Your chronic anxiety is an extremely high form. It's considered a mental condition that makes you feel extremely distressed, frightened, or frightened when you feel comfortable, safe, or safe in normal situations. In such situations, you can become helpless, paralyzed, or even immobilized by such fearful sensations insofar as your normal day-to-day functioning has already been affected. <u>Three of the most frequent anxiety problems are:</u>

* **General Anxiety:** Intense, extreme, and frequently out of this world, and even in the safest and most normal situations, worries.

* **Panic:** Terror feelings that suddenly come frequently and regularly from nowhere. In general, panic attacks are caused by chest pains, abundant sweating, shock, or palpitations. The intensity of these usually increases as someone with panic attacks can feel that they are nuts or have a heart attack.

* **Phobia:** This refers to chronic extreme fear of specific items or situations like insects, aircraft, dark rooms, and boats. Phobias are excessively important because you avoid your life's important daily activities to avoid objects or feared situations.

* **PTSD** – Post-traumatic stress disorder generally occurs when a person has seen or seen traumatic things. Symptoms may start immediately or may appear weeks, months, years later. Some of the most common causes

include war, physical attacks, natural catastrophes, and anxiety episodes.

* **OCD:** Obsessive-compulsive disorder is already regarded as an anxiety disorder, but only recently. People who have OCD usually have to repeat certain rituals, including constantly washing hands, counting, and verifying something repeatedly.

* **Social Anxiety:** A particular type of anxiety is to communicate with individuals – social interactions and circumstances. This extreme sense of fear is usually fuel by worries about being ridiculed, rejected, embarrassed, or simply embarrassed.

Other people are being seen in a negative light. It is what we will talk about in all the rest of this book's chapters.

## Symptoms of Anxiety

So how do you differentiate between anxiety and a normal anxiety disorder? <u>Here are some signs that might suggest you anxiety disorder regularly:</u>

- ✓ **<u>Nights without sleep:</u>** Worrying makes sleep as easy as sprinting 1 kilometer on a steep uphill path or murmuring at a rock concert with your friend. Why does this happen? It's because this sensation raises your heartbeat, which increases your senses as you are already expected to relax.

- ✓ **<u>Sweaty Or Cold feet And Hands:</u>** Because anxiety increases your heart rate, your body pulls more blood into places. It feels more appropriate and decreases blood flow to your extremities, especially your hands and feet. The temperature in these areas appears to decrease due to lower blood flow. The temperature in your hands and feet might be the same as those parts of the body with an elevated blood fluid, and so signal them to sweat as if they were hot. So hands and feet are cold but moist.

✓ **<u>Palpitations:</u>** A highly apparent effect of anxiety is dramatically higher or more rapid. It's a potential sign of an anxiety disorder if it appears to happen excessively and without a sound foundation.

✓ **<u>You feel like you can't breathe:</u>** Anxiety – natural or disorders – causes you to breathe in more air than is common or appropriate. If you do this – hyperventilation – the body has significantly compromised its carbon-oxygen balance, making you believe that you will not obtain adequate oxygen in this overabundance.

✓ **Can't remain still:** All this adrenaline is secreted in an agitated state by your body, making you unrest and restless.

✓ **Nauseous feeling:** if you are nervous, the stress system will turn around and change many things inside the body, such as disturbance of the digestive process of your abdomen, in particular the suppression. When that happens, you feel nauseous or, in the worst-case scenario, puke, one of the undesirable effects.

✓ **Strong muscles:** No, I'm not referring to fitness and muscles. I speak of chronically tensed muscles. I speak because of yourself.

Whenever you're nervous, your body flips on its combat/flight system. This combat-or-flight mechanism prepares your body for unconscious muscle tension to take off or defend itself fastly. It's like getting ready to lift a sprint in a relay run.

- ✓ <u>Mouth parched:</u> Your mouth dries up for many reasons because of anxiety. If you are anxious but unconscious, you tend to breathe in the mouth, and the air that passes through it dries up the saliva. Acid reflux also induces anxiety and dries up your mouth by stopping your salivary drums from generating enough saliva to keep your mouth moist.

## Impact of Anxiety Disorders On Your Body

Anxiety disorders are not laughable as they can have a significant effect on your life. For one thing, these conditions put the body in a constant state of high drive and stress that increase the risk for some of the most serious health problems such as high cholesterol, diabetes, short-term memory loss, issues with the digestive system, heart defects, heart attacks, and poor immune systems.

Anxiety disorders, particularly with a sweet tooth, can significantly increase your risk of diabetes. It is because stressful conditions tend to make you consume foods filled with sugar to deal with. Since your body is in a chronic hyperdrive condition, anxiety disorders tend to consume more calories, making you sense you need more energy and quickly. And imagine what kind of food and beverages will help you quickly to become energized? OK – sugar foods! That's right!

The same applies to your cholesterol risk. Anxiety disorders appear to overstimulate the nervous system by releasing certain hormone forms that can lead to an increased risk of increased cholesterol levels.

Diseases of Anxiety can also impair the capacity of your body to absorb what you eat. Why does this happen? That is because anxiety, which is mainly a mental activity or disease, increases your brain's activity and slows down other vital functions of your body, including the digestion of what you are wolfing.

It raises the risk for diarrhea, bloating, or indigestion digestive issues.

Anxiety disorders could also make you look like Dory, a lovingly forgettable fish in the 2003 hit film Finding Nemo. In the film, Dory had a very pleasant and lovely short-term memory loss. Yet the only thing that makes anxiety look like Dory is the part of forgetfulness, not the cute, lovely parts. Why does this happen? Anxiety increases your cortisol (stress hormone), which can significantly impact your mental performance, particularly memory and reminder.

Also, you can raise the probability of getting sniffs and cough with anxiety issues, among others. If persistent, the immune system appears to be messy with the short- or long-term effect, mainly because of cortisol. And tend to get sick more frequently with a weakened immune system.

Finally, heart disease anxiety disorders can increase the risk. The heart rate and blood pressure can be chronically increased, and both increase the risk of death, particularly because of a heart attack.

## How can your Social life impact Anxiety

Social anxiety and phobia are going to mess with the connections and social experiences. What can be enjoyable and friendly moments would otherwise turn out to be moments of fear and panic, which can separate you from most of the world.

## How anxiety can kill your prospects

You will have to take risks to succeed in life. The higher the success, the higher the risk that you must take. However, Anxiety disorders decrease the risk perception by considerably higher risks than possible rewards. You may be prevented from even attempting to succeed with the risks that seem to be imminent and much greater than the possible benefits.

## Is there a treatment for disorders of anxiety?

Well, the news about the treatment of anxiety disorders is both positive and bad. I'm going to first give you the bad news from my extremely optimistic and friendly heart: no, it can't be cured. The next time you end up with a huckster who offers a remedy against anxiety disorder for your unpredictably low price, it is time to kick some ass and shake up some of your faces. There is a better understanding than to think that a cured solution exists for these home shopping network gadgets' fat loss claims.

Are you ready to know the good one after you've done away with the bad news? It is here: You can manage it effectively so that your ability to live fully does not interfere. Yes, you can manage it so well that it is not a disorder anymore.

## SOCIAL ANXIETY NUTRITIONAL TACTICS

How often did you hear that you're what you're eating? It's true to some degree. You're eating healthy food; you're getting healthy. You eat waste; your body turns into waste. You eat food that will help you to calm down, to calm down.

Eating the right food can improve your ability to manage anxiety greatly and cope with it. Right to eat includes whole foods, herbs, and other food.

## Whole Foods To Enjoy

Regardless of how you say it, it is always healthier for entire food to eat than processed foods, irrespective of the healthy manufacturers. The Paleo Principle is an excellent guiding principle in evaluating how good a food product is or how unhealthy. The closer a food product to its original shape, the better it is. This principle states. Thus it is clear between the apple and the apple piece, which is healthier between the two.

Why is transformed food less than whole foods? With so much processing, including cooking, the most essential and beneficial food nutrients are lost. Worse, some processing processes make food unhealthy either because of changes in the food's molecular structure or because unhealthy ingredients are added. You will have to take all the nutrients you can obtain and minimize unhealthy ingredients if you want to manage your social anxiety very well.

The Mayo Clinic promotes several dietary practices to cope with and manage social anxiety, or just about all anxiety disorders. One of them eats a high-protein breakfast. It'll make you feel full of eating protein for long periods. It also helps to stabilize your blood sugar levels throughout the rest of the morning for stable energy.

Another dietary practice in the Mayo Clinic is complex carbohydrates rather than simple carbohydrates. Carbohydrates can help you manage your social anxiety by encouraging more serotonin production in your brain. Higher serotonin levels are beneficial for anxiety, as you learned earlier. Why is carbohydrates complex? It is because complex carbs help you maintain a stable level of blood sugar, enhancing and alerting you and reducing your risk of diabetes. These are two less worrying things.

Adequate water is another healthy dietary practice that Mayo Clinic pushes to cope with and manage anxiety. Dehydration can affect your mood so that your anxiety is triggered. Go 6 to 8 glasses a day, as a general instruction, and do not wait for your urine to turn dark yellow before gulping on. You're dehydrated by that time already.

Mayo Clinic promotes balanced, healthy meals, which are important for optimal mental health, as are all other nutrition experts. Loading fresh fruits and vegetables in particular and rich in omega-3 fats

For fishes such as salmon and trout, Be aware that you should still be cautious not to over-feed even if you consume healthy and balanced food.

Some of the best foods to eat to manage and cope with your social anxiety – or any general anxiety problems – are:

i.  **Acai berries:** This is another superfood packed with phytonutrients and antioxidants, as with blueberries.

ii.  **Almonds:** The high content of zinc is an excellent reason for this noodle. In maintaining a balanced mood, zinc plays a vital role in reducing fear. It is also high in iron, which is important since the anemia may make you feel more tired than usual. It is also high in iron.

iii.  **Blueberries:** This super dense nutrient packages lots of phytonutrients, antioxidants, and vitamins to combat stress.

iv.  **Chocolates:** Hallelujah! Yeah, you read that correctly. Hold your riding, but I'm not talking of Cadbury, Snickers, and Hershey's commercial versions that are highly processed and full of sugar. The sugar and the dark chocolate without milk is the purest form I'm talking about. The mood enhances pure dark chocolates. It also helps to reduce the level of cortisol. Remember the stress hormone cortisol?

v. **Seaweeds:** A good alternative for whole grains to get enough magnesium and tryptophan.

vi. **Whole grains:** This is very good for you, but only if you are not sensitive to gluten. • Whole grains: Complex carbon for constant energy and tryptophan to produce the soothing hormone serotonin are charged with magnesium (not enough for aggravating anxiety).

## Herbs

Did you know that herbs could also help your social anxiety, apart from making a lot of your dishes even more delicious? One reason is that they are all-natural and so healthy. Secondly, some herbs can manage anxiety. The following herbs are:

i.   **Lavender:** In a 2010 study conducted to manage persistent widespread anxiety disorders, oil extracted from this herb was shown to be as effective as the famous anti-anxiety Benzie Lorazepam. The good part? The good part? The same sedation effects do not occur. How can I use it? Start as aromatherapy for anxiety relief with 80 milligrams daily.

ii.  **Passion Flower:** Studies have found that, according to the University of Maryland Medical Center, this herb works as well as some Benzies to cope and managing anxiety but, as in lavender, less sedation. Another study also demonstrated that it reduces anxiety, restlessness, irritability, and depression in previously recovering opium addicts. How can I use it? Start your 3-fold daily with 90 mg of your fluid extract or a cup of flowers.

iii. **Lemon Balm:** This herb can also help with the management and management of fear on its own, normally used for other herbs. In 2004, a published study showing lemon balm (600 milligrams, to be exact) alerted and calmed participants and reduced stress rates. How can I use it? Start with one tea cubicle with dried lemon balm up to 4 times daily.

iv. **Chamomile Tea:** This is a tea that will not make you more alert but will help you calm down, making handling and administering your social anxiety disorder much easier. It contains positive compounds that imitate the effects of another benzene, valium, which connects to important receptors of your brain. Subjects' anxiety decreased significantly in a study conducted by the University of Pennsylvania following eight weeks of chamomile tea.

v. **Hops:** Sorry, the ingredient itself does not refer to the finished (beer) product. Hop extracts can especially be used for the therapy of flavoring n that your pillows purchase. It is rarely consumed as a tea because of its bitter taste

## Additions

Today, all your daily dietary requirements cannot be obtained solely from food. Most agricultural soil is already tired these days, i.e., over-farming, significantly lower nutritional content. Indeed, people from ages ago appeared to be more knowledgeable than us in recognizing soil fatigue. The Old Testament of the Bible required the Jews not to plant anything on their farmland for one year in seven years.

The storeroom, transport, and transportation across long distances are another reason we cannot get all our nutritional requirements from whole foods, particularly vegetables and fruits. In particular, most foods and vitamins, particularly vitamin B-complex and C, are often removed during long storage periods.

Lastly, the heating meal also destroys nutrients, especially high-temperature cooking. Since it is highly unlikely that all nuts can be produced from foods that are not called sushi and sashimi for most people, it is very unlikely.

Do you want to know how unfeasible it is to obtain important vitamins and minerals with all your recommended daily allowance (RDA)? Take Vitamin E, with approximately 30 IU or global units in the RDA. <u>You will have to eat this much every day for you to get this from food:</u>

- ❖ 10 pounds or 40 ears of fresh maize on average;

- ❖ 2 pounds of the sprout of wheat

- ❖ Three pounds of almonds

- ❖ Spinach of 33 pounds

- ❖ Broccoli 50 pounds.

When you anticipate that you cannot eat that much in one day, consider that it's only for vitamin E alone. How about the vitamins and minerals that are other important? As early as now, I can say that your tummy would explode if you tried it!

Now that I have made a case for supplements, here are a few supplements that can help you control social concerns properly:

- ✓ **Gamma-Amino Butyric Acid:** Also known for its brevity as GABA, there is evidence of its capacity to improve rest. As such, it is supposed to help manage the symptoms of anxiety.

- ✓ **Kava:** The most prevalent and popular management of anxiety

Market supplement. It may also have the most scientific support. Studies have shown that some of the most common prescription anxiety medicines on the market are cumbersome. Even as a supplement, the prescription medicines are similar in that they are not well mixed with alcohol and other prescription medications. Also, if you had a history of liver or alcoholic disease, recover, or still have one, you can do well to avoid this. But even if you are clear about this and this is not pharmaceutical grade, you would be well advised to get clearance first for your doctor.

❖ **<u>Magnesium:</u>** Not getting sufficient magnesium is widely believed to cause or exacerbate anxiety symptoms such as panic or social anxiety. Magnesium is important for healthy nerves and can influence the levels of anxiety.

❖ **<u>Melatonin:</u>** This sleep-inducing hormone is considered an anxiety control aid with good potential, which is naturally occurring in your body. It can help relieve some of your anxiety because it relaxes your body. Please be careful. However, in some areas, melatonin needs a prescription, so be sure that you have one if in a place where it is required. It can also make you sleep, especially at higher dosages, against your wishes. Therefore, make sure that you begin with half the smallest possible dosage to measure tolerance.

❖ **Passionflower:** This herb is also available as a nutritional supplement. While not as powerful as Kava, it reacts to alcohol and is generally good for managing anxiety levels.

❖ **Valerian Root:** the additional form of this herb-inducing sleep can help you relax and manage your social anxiety. Some studies have validated the ability to improve anxiety symptoms.

❖ **Vitamin B12:** This vitamin is essential to a healthy nervous system, just like magnesium. Some studies have also shown that adding vitamin B12 to your diet can improve your anxiety symptoms.

## Supplementary Caution

Although you are not considered a drug and therefore do not need any prescriptions, you would do well to consult your doctor before taking any of these supplements. Better safe than sorry because these can hinder your ability, especially if you are suffering from a medical condition or take other prescription medicines or supplements. Prevention is always better than treatment.

## How to create an anti-anxiety diet

We can't blame you for food for your anxiety. But what you eat and how you eat helps you manage fear. Some foods are 'designed' to cause anxiety symptoms, while others can help you cope with them.

Diet matters, but it's a vicious cycle. Many who are anxious are going to eat comfort food to make them feel better. But what you ingest has a direct impact on your feelings and your anxiety levels

– High sugar, high carbohydrate foods make you feel better, but just for a few minutes, while other foods release certain sensational chemicals. The right balance can be a useful tool for coping with the symptoms of a social anxiety disorder.

We all have heard the term "healthier eating," which has been thrown a little over these days, but it makes a difference to eat a healthier diet when it comes to anxiety. When you fill your plate with vegetables, your anxiety symptoms will combat better than an unhealthy burger plate.

The way to create an anxiety diet is to remove certain foods – which can be very good for the symptoms of your anxiety. **The following foods should be removed or minimized:**

- Fried foods are extremely hard to digest, very little in nutrition, and contribute to a risk of cardiovascular disease. You will fight to combat anxiety symptoms if your body can not properly handle the food you are eating

- Alcohol – several individuals with an anxiety disorder turn to alcohol in the wrong conviction that it will improve everything. That's not the case. Although too many things can make you stupid, alcohol does not benefit your body. It dehydrates, discards the balance of your hormones, and it also strikes your nutritional balance. And physical anxiety symptoms can result from the toxins that enter your body.

- Coffee-Caffeine is a stimulant and will not, in moderation, cause any problems with symptoms of anxiety. The more you consume, however, the worse the risk. Coffee also helps your heart to beat faster and also to make you feel more panicked. Limit your daily consumption to one cup.

- Dairy-Dairy products are not bad for you, as long as you ingest them in moderation. Large quantities of milk can increase your adrenaline levels and contribute to increased anxiety.

Decrease the amount you eat, cut it down, or cut it completely if you find that eating milk causes your symptoms to worsen.

- Refined Sugar – While fruit sugar is not bad, dessert sugar is bad. Like caffeine, sugar stimulates the human body to produce some shakiness, which can exacerbate your anxiety symptoms.

- Food That Forms Acid - The acid in the body is made of yogurt, eggs, pickles, wine, sour cream, and liver, and there are good grounds to think that the magnesium level is also reduced in the body. Low magnesium is one of the causes or contributors to fear, especially in those who have an anxiety disorder, so it is wise to cut back or off the food.

It can certainly help you avoid these types of foods, but you will not cure your anxiety disorder, especially if you find that you eat over one or more of them.

You don't have to eat a rabbit diet; most foods can still be consumed, but moderation is important if you help reduce anxiety symptoms. Remember this – a nutritionally sound body is better capable than one filled with junk foods to combat symptoms.

## 6 Types of food to help you combat anxiety

So you know what to avoid, but you know what to eat more? The following nutrients can help reduce anxiety symptoms. A healthy diet helps your hormones work correctly and leads to a general sense of well-being. **Try incorporating these foods into your diet:**

- **Fresh fruit** – but the body does not need the refined, needs a certain amount of sugar and carbon hydrates. The fresh fruit contains natural sugars that are burned down and transformed into energy. They also include nutrients, including vitamins and antioxidants, which are necessary. Blueberries and fishing are the best two.

- **Vegetables** - The vegetables, particularly if you have an anxiety disorder, are even more essential than fruit. Most vegetables contain high fiber levels and are filled with vitamins, particularly with anxiety disorders, which are rapidly depleted.

- **Water** - Most people are dehydrated because they don't drink enough water anywhere. Dehydration places the body in anxiety and can make fighting the symptoms much harder. Try to drink a minimum of 1 l/15 to 2 l/d/day.

- **Tryptophan-rich food** - These foods have proven to be extremely effective in helping to reduce anxiety symptoms. They include a component that helps you relax naturally, which is always a bonus and can also increase your metabolism—foods such as poultry, soy, sésame, and oats.

- **Foods rich in magnesium**—approximately 25% of the population is magnesium deficient and a nutrient that plays a significant part in the body. Magnesium is involved in over three hundred different body processes is essential to get adequate amounts of them. Magnesium is rich in foods such as tofu and black beans.

- **Omega-3 Fatty Acids** – We know a nutrient vital to anxiety and depression while research in omega-3 Fatty acids is still ongoing. Fatty fish, like salmon and mackerel, winter squash, and flaxseed, can produce omega-3s.

**THE MINDFULNESS**

## NATURE OF YOUR TRUE MIND

We have many thoughts, and they all move around with what we are aware of. Just as identical objects will each contain different characteristics, they will each experience the object differently. As opposed to a tree for a botanist, a carpenter has a different way of viewing the same tree.

Our many senses cloud each other, but they are all the same. These phenomena call the ocean; each one reacts differently. Ours is just one of many minds that there are. They are a part of the society that always converges and moves to entertain themselves or for enjoyment. In the One True Mind, which does not move, it is fully settled, and the universe, which is moving, revolves around it as it observes all that goes and does not move.

We perceive the mind as a free-floating, ever-changing cloud of associations, events, and experiences. It is not an essential, defining feature of us as individuals. Instead, it is the vast majority of our broader past that we bring with us into each new cognitive state. Furthermore, when we die, the mind dies along with the body. But actually, a different kind of mind has already taken shape.

If we try to locate the One True Mind, we will never find it. As the Buddha said in one very excellent discourse, if our mind were inside our body, it would be aware of things inside the body, our fingers, and such. After all, the mind does the feeling; just because the body is inside, our mind does not mean that our mind reflects directly on the body. If it were outside your body, like the phone you are pointing at now, it would see your face. We know that it is neither inside your body nor outside. The true mind is in nature; it doe s not move; it is not fixed; it is not locatable, nor is it graspable. The true nature of your mind is quite unimaginable, though.

There is an interesting tale about a person who was told to love and be truly devoted to the Prophet Mohammed. He contemplated this but loving someone that lived a thousand years ago wouldn't have been possible to do. He told his teacher, "Exactly!" After thinking about it, he realized he meant something else.

As you can infer from above, this is the true nature of mind, God, or any level of ultimate truth, even true love. It is so unimaginable. You cannot think it, you will not understand it, and you cannot explain it. This [subject] is beyond the nature of your logical mind. It is not for you to experience. It is the place where the koans are made to apply logic, an unanswerable riddle that is meant to torture the mind until it gives up logical thought.

In his book "Tao Te Ching," Lao Tzu looks to the idea that 'The Tao that is be named is not the eternal Tao.' Either it cannot be conceived or explained in any other way than by the kind of knowledge you can only obtain by being one of the limited numbers of minds. How can anyone think of or imagine an unlimited being? That is not possible because there is only one God, no matter which name you give, but only one reality about a tree's toughness as you constantly seek to grasp the truth, whose only Ultimate Truth is. Make sure that you understand that [in the case of the nature of your True Mind], you cannot understand it and only experience it. And this can only be done by stopping all mental activity by standing still or stilling your mind with the realization and realization of your present state of mind's falsity. When someone says that their personal feeling or belief is "the truth" and that yours is "total falsity," that person lives in complete false beliefs. Since in the language, "truth" means something the speaker believes is true at that specific moment, there is only one truth, which is one of many perspectives about that one truth.

To achieve this realization is the goal of spiritual work. Active thinking is a great tool, but users should be aware that it is like a melon or nut's skin. The skin protects the fruit by putting up a barrier over the fruit, and once the fruit is ripe, it is discarded. A rational mind seems to believe that the very thing that is most difficult is also the most valuable. We use it to ponder the nature of the One True Mind, but there comes the point where we must discard any ideas that we have developed about it. However, progress can be made without discriminatory, higher thinking processes, but we have not yet revealed why this is rarely the case.

If that is true, we do not need to find the One True Mind because we believe that our discriminating mind is our true mind, and that is a lie. We believe a lie because we do not have any way of knowing better. Our minds get fooled into thinking other people are the real mind because they are not aware of all the individual's mind and body's distractions and weaknesses. We can see each mind's limited nature in our study and self-observation of the nature of discriminating minds belonging to every sense and in many parts of us than we know. We return to the idea of a path to enlightenment and freedom, emphasizing removing obstacles rather than acquiring more knowledge.

You can begin to see the difference between the discriminating mind and One True Mind if you can achieve a momentary experience of the true nature of your mind, the solidity of the mind that is not either inside or outside of your being.

## EXERCISE

Rest at a crossroads outside. Look at the middle of the crossroads, on the floor. Don't take a peek and let both cars and pedestrians pass by without turning your head from one point you're attached to. Don't tighten your eyes; just let your eyes look at it.

Note the sounds and smells and the sights critically. Without attention, let everything go by. Enable your mind to rest on a certain spot without consideration about something you feel, and hold your breath and eyes focused on one spot, then remember this lesson. Sit in one place and let the world pass by. Feel your mind, feeling mind, and smelling mind. Notice your mind. Note how many minds you have and how they all tear from your One True Mind at your attention.

## The lesson is going on now.

You must first demonstrate that you have many minds and believe that they are your One True Mind before you can even allow yourself to encounter the mind's true character. It is done by remembering how many times, without you realizing it, you are about one topic and another. Right now, you can show that by trying to place all your concentration 5 minutes in your left hand. Feel the air temperature around your palm, the texture of everything it affects, and all other sensations that your hand has without a gap of consciousness for a strong 5 minutes. How could you profess a unified mind or your life in general control or awareness for just a few minutes? Maybe you have a second-hand analog clock or look. Try to keep your second hand completely concentrated for seven minutes without drifting into another thought; even try for a minute.

Yourself-will is the essence of your true mind and cannot be pushed anywhere it wishes to be. You can stay focused on what you choose for as long as you touch with your true mind. To begin work on it, we need evidence of any definition, and if you do not show it and believe in the evidence, you will be unable to move on. You might find it so devastating to turn your head away quickly and to revive your former life as autumn.

Now, if the true mind is not inside or without you, where is that? What? It can only be everywhere if it is neither here nor there. That's how mental abilities work. You're not going to one place or another. You're already there that isn't moving or a certain specified position, thus anywhere in the actual mind nature. At the same time, here and there.

## **EXERCISE**

Look at a skyscraper or mountain. Let your mind ponder the notion that your true mind is all at once everywhere. It's like the various atoms in the universe. It's all around and thus all.

Just let your mind relax while you transfer your Tai Chi core. You were told to bring your focus into one part of the body, note it in your head, then take it to your throat, chest, lower it, lower it, and then go back up.

It is where your center is relocated. Do this when you look at or pick the mountain or the house. It settles your mind in one place and starts to perceive the essence of your real and immovable mind by gathering your ideas and holding them in one place instead of allowing them to travel all over the world. You make the whole of the universe one thing, and in one viewpoint, you'd look at several things. You could find that you are not as limited as you feel if you can find your core in your sound mind and look at an outdoor object. It is an activity to which the guide will guide you but does not lead you.

Zen archery, Kyudo, is a very good sport. You look at the goal and don't concentrate on anything else as you faithfully track every aspect of your body.

## Return to the lecture.

Therefore, we have determined that the real essence of your mind is not what you interpret and recognize as your mind or being. If something is moving and you see its motion, what is moving? It's the moving stuff, not your simple mind. You will start to relax in your One True Mind if you can stabilize your many minds by understanding how they take you as a dog along with a leash in tandem with all of the phenomena of the universe. Only by faithfully believing the lies you believe in yourself, in particular by knowing what you are and knowing the nature of your mind, can you conclude that there is only one truth, and you can only start work. It's not the flag waving in the wind until then or the wind which moves it, but the intellect.

There is just one truth saying that the various realities people pretend to have are only delusions. Everything you feel is only a subjective illusion of one of the many moving minds that move you away from the single, unmoving, true mind. Fighting what you believe in is like hanging on the anchor of an ocean ship or defending your beliefs and opinions.

You can not experience the essence of your true mind if you do not give up the idea of something you understand because it is, as we said, impossible. You forbid that the mind is blank and silent, the only way to experience the existence of the One True Mind.

You believe, or you have little knowledge of truth or fact. If you hold a lie to be true, you cannot find the truth.

Funny enough, you will have absolute awareness if you let go of your false view of reality, including that of your thought or the illusion that you believe you do not know your mind (both equal trixters) since you have reached the One True Mind which is everywhere.

The journey will take several years. As you advance, you may develop those skills step by step, but you should never be warned that you have reached the full degree of understanding of the One True Mind because, in the shadow, there will always be a writer. You'll know when you get them, and you can't describe them or identify them.

Be the rock in the turbulence, don't move. It sounds so complicated, and you're probably right. You're not sure. You or any human being would possibly be unable to achieve perfect illumination. However, the state of your being can be changed very much. Don't get frustrated because you can see the big challenge ahead and make it your destination and try to get as near as you can. One more phase is yet another. Better to be shifted by a little stone than a destroyed leaf.

## Staying in the Present

If you've read some kind of mindfulness books or done some meditation, you've probably heard of staying in the present. At first, this might seem a bit stupid, and you might think, How can I be anywhere but the present? Right now, I'm here. I'm freaking out here right now because I think I might have touched something I wasn't supposed to touch an hour ago. I mean, in a week or two, I'm going to figure out that I caught a disease! Just now, it's awful! But that's not right now. It is the twisted version of your OCD right now. It is the past that no longer exists and the future that exists only in theory. In other words, it is the "what if" in which OCD lives, not the "what is," o material for the OCD to work within the "what is." You're just a person reading a book, looking at the words right now. In the present, even thinking can be done. Okay, you're a person who's thinking. There's nothing there to get the OCD's claws into. However, in "what if," there is a fear of what might have happened or what might still have happened. Then there is the urge to do something about that fear, to keep it from being realized. It is a compulsion. Another way to see this is to acknowledge that mindfulness keeps your mind close to your body. With this book, your body is sitting in a chair. Your mind is with you, reading these words. When your mind wanders to replay a conversation you had last week or think about an upcoming event, your mind is nowhere near your body. In that space, OCD assumes ownership of the mind. Can you think of a moment when, instead of remaining where you are at the moment, you sometimes find your mind traveling to the past or the future? Accepting what is going on right now, being truly mindful does not necessarily mean feeling at peace. You might feel anxious right now. What this may mean is that right now, where you sit, as you are, you don't know when or if the thoughts, feelings, and sensations you're experiencing will ever go away. You can look at it without judgment only in the present and potentially experience it without fear.

## Thoughts Are Thoughts, Not Threats

It is not just the content of thoughts that make the primary difference, but their perspective on thoughts. If you think that particular thinking is "bad" in itself, this may be a problem. A series of factors may influence the way a thought is "bad." If you are in a fully relaxed state, it might seem unworthy to consider snapping and doing something crazy. The same thinking might seem like an awful accusation or a warning of coming to a nightmare in an anxious state. I need to get that out if it is in my mind! When people with OCD and other anxiety disorders can imagine that their thoughts are like train buses, they tend to stop the train to make sure everyone gets a ticket. Pay attention to the fact that you just watch the train as it passes. You're just on your way to work at the station. You don't have to take part in tickets and ensure that the right people are on the correct trains. It means recognizing that unwanted thoughts take place but not assessing them as particularly significant. Instead of changing the thinking, you change your perspective to the thinking and how you proceed with the thinking. It doesn't happen to you. It's just going on.

## Thoughts as Words

The idea that ideas are thoughts, not threats, is also considered by looking at how you perceive words. You call it what it concerns when you see a word. Steven Hayes (2005) describes how the mind consists of a network of "relational frames" with concepts experienced internally as they relate to in his excellent workbook Get Out of Your Mind and Into Your Life. When you feel an OCD thought, you are also conscious of all the things you refer to. You don't have any problem with many thoughts, but you perceive obsession as something of greater value than thoughts, feelings, and sensations associated with your disorder. It's all the stuff you associate with, not just an obsession. Practice: This is a practice when you see how the mind works. See the words below.

## MIRROR

Ask yourself, what does that mean? Well, this is a mirror. It's a mirror. It is a mirror, right. Right. However, we would consider this a bit odd if you stared at this page and tried to make your hair or makeup by using it. In the previous mirror, you do not see your reflection. It isn't a mirror, therefore. The word "speaker" is it. But is the word "speaker?" Yes and no. "M-I-R-R-O-R" is a string of lyrics in a specific order, which gives us the idea of a text called a "mirror," a reflective surface of the glass. We call it a word. "MIRROR" means little. And anyway, what are letters?

We have agreed to give a certain value, only symbols, small drawings. It's an "M," a "R," etc. It is an "M." Thus, several symbols without meaning are given meaning and then placed in an order that adds meaning. This set of symbols is referred to as a "word," which triggers an idea. In this case, this idea generates images of a reflective surface and all related thoughts, feelings, and sensations, which accompany a consciousness of being close to a reflective surface. If you are OCD, you opened this book, and a mirror fell to the floor. The ideas are shown to be intrinsically valuable, automatic, and urgently relevant to a certain behavioral response. The practice of carefulness suggests you look at the thought as you look at words. They are empty vessels, which are empowered and looked upon by the mind. The idea of contamination is not the same as contamination. It is thought of it. It's a thought.

## SELF LOVE

## WHAT IS SELF-LOVE?

Self-love is a condition of appreciation for oneself that develops from activities that help our physical, mental and spiritual development. Self-love means having high respect for your prosperity and joy. Self-love means dealing with your necessities and not forfeiting your capital to satisfy others. Self-love means not agreeing to short of what you merit.

Self-love can mean something else for every individual since we have a wide range of approaches to deal with ourselves. Sorting out what self-love resembles for you as an individual is a significant piece of your psychological wellness. I've accounted for self-love 3ly: purpose, self-esteem, and spirit. These are every component of self-love.

- **Purpose:** You understand what you're acceptable at, what your abilities and blessings are, and you need to utilize them to improve the world. You realize you have something to give, and you WANT to share it. It's cheerful for you to give it. Living with purpose causes you to feel alive, meaningful, huge, and loved.

- **Self-esteem:** You feel SECURE IN WHO YOU ARE. Certain. Not any more self-analysis and unforgiving judgment. All things being equal, you have sympathy for yourself and persistence with yourself. You anticipate that yourself should be great. However, you're ready to be straightforward with yourself. The old uncertainties you've been hauling around for quite a long time are at last supplanted with feeling free from any harm on the planet and inside yourself.

- **Spirit:** Our feeling of spirit is regarding our actual, spiritual nature. You feel straightforwardly associated with something more significant, cherishing, and health of your most elevated tremendous, and most prominent recuperating. We are intended to love ourselves for some reasons, however mainly, so we can make the world a kinder spot.

## WHAT DOES SELF-LOVE LOOK LIKE?

Coming up next are instances of what self-love can resemble in real life.

- ✓ Directing positive sentiments toward yourself

- ✓ Pardoning yourself when you jumble up

- ✓ Addressing your requirements

- ✓ Being confident

- ✓ Don't allow others to exploit or maltreat you.

- ✓ Focusing on your wellbeing and prosperity

- ✓ Investing energy around individuals who uphold you and develop you (and staying away from individuals who don't)

- ✓ Requesting help

- ✓ Relinquishing feelings of spite or outrage that keeps you down

- ✓ Perceiving your qualities

- ✓ Esteeming your feelings

- ✓ Settling on reliable decisions more often than not

- ✓ Living as per your qualities

- ✓ Seeking after your inclinations and objectives.

- ✓ Testing yourself

- ✓ Considering yourself responsible

- ✓ Giving yourself solid treats

- ✓ Tolerating your blemishes

- ✓ Setting reasonable assumptions

- ✓ Seeing your advancement and exertion

**PART B**

# FOCUSING ON YOUR GOALS.

## <u>Goal-Setting</u>

### <u>What is goal setting?</u>

The procedure of taking active actions to achieve your wanted result is goal-setting. Your dream may be to become an instructor, a musician, or a physical therapist. Each of these dreams includes setting small (and big!) goals and achieving them. It is possible to break down each of these primary goals into smaller, more achievable goals that will propel you towards success.

<u>There are three kinds of goals-goals of process, performance, and result.</u>

- Process targets are specific performance actions or 'processes.' For example, to study every day for 2 hours after dinner. Process priorities are 100 percent controllable by the person.

- Goals for performance are based on personal standards. They are aiming to achieve a 3.5 GPA, for example. Mostly, individual objectives are controllable.

- Outcome objectives are based on winning. It could seem like landing a job in your field for a college student or landing a job at a specific employment place you wanted. Because of other external influences, outcome targets are challenging to control.

The goals of process, performance, and result have a linear relationship. It is important because you give yourself an excellent opportunity to accomplish your performance goals if you achieve your process objectives. Similarly, you have a better chance of achieving your outcome target when you reach your performance goals.

## What are the Tips for General Goal Setting?

➤ Set both short- and long-term objectives

- Set SMART objectives

- Set priorities that motivate you

- Jot down your objectives and place them in a place where you can see

- Adjust your objectives as necessary,

- When you meet a goal, recognize and reward yourself.

## Set SMART targets

Set all three types of objectives-process, performance, and result-but concentrate on achieving your smaller process goals to give you the best chance of success!

i. Specific, highly comprehensive statement on what you want to achieve (use who, what, where, how, etc.)

ii. Measurable- How are you going to show and evaluate how your goal has been achieved?

iii. Achievable-they can be accomplished through your hard work and commitment-ensure that your goals are within your ability to accomplish

iv.   Relevant: How do your goals align with your goals?

v.    Time-based-set 1 or more target dates- these are the "by when to guide the successful and timely completion of your goal (include deadlines, frequency, and dates)

## Why is Goal Setting Important?

Picture this In a metropolis, you are lost and are entirely clueless on which way to go, with so many confusing paths adding to your confusion. A GPS device is the only device that can bail you out of this. Well, in your life, goal setting serves as a GPS, keeping you on the right path towards your destination and saving you from aimless wandering. "Goals are the fuels in the furnace of accomplishment," Brian Tracy once said. An act of goal-setting itself can be signified as the point of embarking on the journey towards one's accomplishments. Having a definite objective allows you to concentrate all of your energies on achieving it. Even your powerful subconscious is stirred when you make a conscious decision to perform a specific purpose. It begins to devise ideas and develop strategies to lead your ambition to fruition. To discover a few of the most important benefits of personal goal setting, reviewed the write-up below.

## What are the Benefits Of Goal Setting?

### It helps you to remain focused

We all yearn to reach great heights in life, but how many of us end up doing it? Possibly, very few. The main reason behind this is that many individuals shed focus on the path and also thus stumble. The most significant importance of setting goals is that it helps you stay focused to achieve what you are looking for. It functions as a steering wheel that moves you in the right direction. The key is the focus. You can't afford, in any way, to take your eyes off the target for even a moment. Setting goals helps you stay focused on life's goals. You can also ensure that your efforts are adequately channelized by dint of practical goal setting, and your faculties are not squandered dealing with mere trifles.

## Assists in procrastination overcoming

Setting objectives also helps you to overcome procrastination. One of the greatest frailties of human nature is the habit of procrastination, which severely jeopardizes one's chances of progress. If you have a set goal for yourself, though, you will always be on the ball and do as needed to accomplish it. On insignificant or unproductive actions, you will waste less time and take a more direct route to achieve the objective.

## Measures progress of yours

The setting of goals works as a measuring measure of your progress that allows you to assess your progress from time to time. You'll have a clear idea of what you've been able to accomplish so far, what you're missing, or how you can improve yourself. You can devise ways to eradicate them and facilitate your progress to achieve the ultimate goal that you have set for yourself once you discern all your shortcomings.

## Sets Obstacles

It allows you to create obstacles. For yourself, setting clear, concrete goals gives you a firm fenceline. To accelerate your progress towards achieving your goal, it creates an invisible barrier, where you decide what you want, what freedoms you have, and what distractions you need to get rid of. It also induces some sense of self-responsibility. You will be obligated to take action instead of just talking about what you want all the time without doing what you need to do to accomplish it. When you first set your goal setting a specific goal clarifies whether you live up to what you committed yourself to do.

## Enables your time to be managed

You will be able to manage your time to your maximum benefit by setting goals. You will have a clear idea of what you have to accomplish in a specific frame of time. Thus all your energy and focus can be channeled towards achieving it. One primary goal can be split into several short-term goals bound by certain time limits, which will make the task easier. It increases the diversity of productivity and effectiveness.

## Motivates

Motivation is an essential ingredient that increases one's chance of achieving one's milestones. Assigning yourself to some short-term objectives will help you achieve them in less time and give you an additional sense of accomplishment that can motivate you to perform better. Once inspired, you will set higher and higher limits for yourself, and, in due time, you will achieve more and more As you begin to live your life with passion, you will experience an upsurge in your energy levels. You will control your life and the direction in which you are headed. Your life will not be determined by fate alone anymore. With your objectives, you create your destiny.

## Stress-Free Life

Your existence can be more organized by a clear objective and an effective game plan. You will be well aware of your concerns by having a clear goal in your mind, and with an efficient time management technique, you will certainly have the ability to achieve your objectives with little effort. You will likewise be without any mental stress, which will further boost your efficiency and productivity.

In the article above, some of the most fruitful benefits of goal setting have been compiled. It is quite clear that the set of objectives is a critical instrument that promotes the prospect of your personal or professional progress. Every goal ought to be concrete and specific. Identifying what you strive for and committing yourself wholeheartedly to achieving it is very important.

# Ways in a world full of distractions to stay focused

The longest chapter in every success story is one about determination.

While success demands many things from us, there is always willpower and determination at the top of the list. Many people think that we are born with determination, and those who succeed are simply the lucky ones who are born with an abundant supply. But if you ask any successful individual, they will tell you that they were not born with more determination; and always found a way of harnessing and using what they got more efficiently.

Here are ways to harness and stay focused on your determination:

- **Set your day up the night before**

Make some fundamental decisions regarding what you're going to do tomorrow before you go to rest, such as what you're going to wear, what you're going to eat for lunch, and the course you're most likely to require to work. The night before, it is easier to pack a healthy lunch than to decide what you will have with a hot dog vendor parked in front of your workplace.

When it comes to spending money, the same applies. Decide and stick to it on a budget.

The night before you check your e-mails or surf the net, decide before you finish the most critical tasks that need to be completed. Stick to your schedule and close your eyes for a few minutes at the end of the day and take in how good you feel about being in charge of your day.

Getting into the habit of scheduling your day in advance will remove your most comfortable choices from the table, making it easier to avoid sidetracking and wasting time and energy on small, unimportant things.

- **Do the most challenging things first**

The more we fret about them or put them off, the more challenging tasks will not get more comfortable. We're only going to waste energy that would be better spent just by digging in. Right away, get after the most challenging job while you are still fresh and have the power.

Research has revealed that our minds are sharpest in the early morning when we must attend to the uphill. We can relax and take care of the more routine work that doesn't require much mental strain, ability, and energy after these are out of the way.

- **Distractions and time-wasters eliminate**

There will be real emergencies, and we need to deal with them. The majority of situations that distract us are not emergencies and do not require us to react immediately. With time, many of these situations will solve themselves on their own.

Responding immediately to these requests will only set you up to receive more. You send a message by not responding that you are a strong-willed, focused individual who is very busy, and you will be less bothered by trivial, time-wasting matters over time.

- **REGENERate and maintain your energy**

When working on something, take a quick break if you feel your energy fading. To take a brief retreat from the job and regenerate, take a brisk walk, run, stretch, or do whatever generates results for you. With renewed vigor and a sharper mental focus, you will come back to your task.

Snack on healthy foods like fresh fruit and vegetables during the day instead of eating a large meal at lunch. Consume great deals of water and enter a regular program of workout. With these things, arrange a routine, so you don't have to think about them; they just become part of your daily regime.

- **Remind yourself always of the ultimate goals**

Create a vision board, a film of the mind, or a system that continually reminds you of what you are working towards. As it will serve as a motivator, the why" behind the goal is crucial.

Suppose that starting a school in a third-world country is why you want to earn $10 million. Have a clear vision of what the school would look like so that you can regularly imagine it. To visualize this objective, set aside regular daily time, if only five minutes. The more specifics that you can put in, the better. By placing music, videos, or anything that gives you an emotional charge, you become emotionally involved with the visualization. It is essential to have an emotional connection, encouraging you to keep moving towards your goal.

## How can your focus be the gateway to your business potential?

In the business world, focus doesn't get the respect it deserves. We hear a lot about motivation, stress, feelings, leadership, and team culture, but the role that focuses on your ability to be productive is not given much attention. Well, I'm here to change that whole thing.

First, let's start with what concentration is. Simply put, the focus includes paying attention to things that will assist and prevent distractions that will harm your work efforts. For example, you need to focus on the relevant data and analyses that will comprise the report to complete a piece. Typical distractions, such as e-mails, being hungry or tired, or the people around you, must also be avoided.

## Without focus, You Can't Think

Focus is essential because it is the gateway to all thinking: understanding, memory, learning, thinking, problem-solving, and decision-making. All facets of your capacity to think will experience without excellent focus. You will not be as efficient in your job without stress because if you do not concentrate on the right things or are distracted, you will not get your job done.

Without adequate focus, you will also not be maximally efficient because you waste time every time your mind wanders away from your job. Finally, because your work output will not be of the highest quality and it will take you longer to do it, you won't be as productive as you can.

Here's a simple reality: you can't think if you can't focus efficiently. And if you can't believe efficiently, you certainly can't produce the quality of work needed to succeed. From this perspective, it is simple to see why the emphasis is vital for business success.

## Progression of Focus

Here's a way you can think of focusing on your work, what I call 'focus progression.' If you concentrate carefully on your work for the time needed without distraction, you will do the necessary work. You will complete the job and produce a quality product in the shortest amount of time if you do the required work in a concentrated way.

## How to Better Focus

The main question is, how can you ensure that you have an ideal work focus that results in productive and effective outputs? <u>Here are a few simple steps:</u>

- <u>De-clutter your mind.</u> One thing you would agree with, I'm sure, is that a cluttered mind can't concentrate. You won't focus well if your mind is filled with things, such as all of the things you need to do today. So, go through and prioritize your assignments. There are things on your calendar that you can either postpone to another day, delegate or not do in all if you resemble many business individuals. Also, clear your mind of anything not related to your job, such as family stuff (of course, easier said than done). The less clutter in your mind, the better you'll be able to concentrate.

It is also not uncommon for business people to have cluttered offices that include myriad photos, books, assorted tchotchkes, a desk filled with junk, not to mention a flat panel on the wall that is always on.

- <u>Create a focused workspace</u>. A clutter-filled workspace means a mind filled with distractions. Simplify your office by removing unnecessary clutter to help you concentrate better. Sure, to make your office an inviting place for you to work, you can keep some family photos and mementos. Remove everything that does not perform a specific job and the crap accumulated on your desk and shelves over the years. Bottom line: a simple workspace is a workspace that is more focused and less distracted.

- <u>Master your technology:</u> In this digital age, the single biggest obstacle to focusing is your technology, including computers, tablets, and smartphones. A constant source of distraction is the pings, vibrations, and other notifications that tell you that a voice mail, e-mail, text message, or social media update has arrived. Two things about so-called multitasking have been demonstrated by recent research. First, the worst multitaskers are people who say they are great multitaskers (as most business people believe they are). Second, at least not when it comes to working; there is no such thing as multitasking. Perhaps the best thing you can do to concentrate is to turn off your technology and focus on the task at hand without distraction or interruption when it's time to get work done.

- <u>Focus on the 4 Ps:</u> Perform the first P. For example, when you are going to start a project, a sales report, strategic plan, marketing analysis, or financial projection, ask yourself what you need to do your best and then create an atmosphere that will allow optimal performance. The second P is a process that involves concentrating entirely on what you need to do to finish a high-quality item without worrying about the outcome. The third P is present, which indicates focusing not on what has occurred in the previous or what might occur in the future yet on the present moment. Finally, the fourth P is the efficiency that only focuses on those things and blocks distractions that allow you to be the most productive you can be.

You have offered a powerful tool that allows you to carry out your work at an ongoingly high level, both useful and reliable if you can control your ability to concentrate. And hinder interruptions, resulting in better quality work, tremendous success, and the achievement of your professional goals.

## Are you proven strategies for overcoming distractions?

There we've all been. Even with the most effective intents to remain on task, we still catch ourselves scrolling via social media sites when we should be working on a mission. The moment we hear a notification, we can not help but grab our cell phone. And there's an e-mail then! If we don't check it every five minutes, we're worried that something important might be missing.

It can seem impossible to avoid distractions. Statistics show that there is a massive productivity loss from distractions. Every 8 mins, the typical manager is disturbed, and employees usually invest 28% of their time handling unnecessary disturbances and trying to come back on track.

So how can you repossess control of your attention and also time?

<u>Seven proven strategies to overcome distractions and reclaim your focus are here.</u>

a.      In distraction-free mode, put yourself.

Start creating habits that allow you to remove distractions and stay focused. Start by creating an atmosphere where you are less tempted to worry about something other than working on. It's not always easy to do this. For one thing, to do our job, many of us rely on a computer, but we also find our biggest distractions enabled by using a computer on the internet. Try using a website blocker app if you permanently find yourself wandering over to video or shopping websites.

Work to create habits that signal that you are in the distraction-free mode to yourself and those around you. Close your office door. Put on headphones for noise-canceling. Switch your phone off or silently put it on and move it away from you so you can't pick it up quickly). You may find it useful to move to a quieter location if you work in an open office. Studies have found that in an open office, distractions happen 64 percent more often, and we are interrupted more often by others in that environment.

Remove as several justifications and also diversions as you can to ensure that one job each time can be brought to your full focus-- no multitasking.

b.        Every day, establish three main goals.

It can feel insurmountable and leave us feeling overwhelmed by a long list of things to do. Before we start, we're ready to give up, and that's when it becomes easy to give in to distractions. By giving yourself three goals to achieve every day, you can offset this. Compose them on a sticky note and also upload them whenever you seek them out from your job, where you can see them.

You'll have specified what you require to work with by limiting the number of daily objectives. You will work with the greater intention on those tasks, and your mind will be less apt to stray.

Ask yourself each morning: What are the three most important things to achieve today? It will help if you put any other assignments on a separate to-do list. Once you've completed the first three goals, you can start to tackle those less-important tasks.

c.      Give yourself a shorter time frame.

More hours worked doesn't mean that more things are necessarily accomplished. The law of Parkinson says that "work tends to expand to fill the time we have available for its completion." And the thing is, we usually fill with distractions any time remaining. It is because, whenever possible, our mind is wired to conserve energy. If there's something we don't have to do, there's a good chance we won't do it. Instead, we'll allow ourselves to get sucked on our phone into a YouTube video or a game app.

On the other hand, we suddenly develop a laser-like focus when we're up against a deadline and avoid distractions at all costs. When you know that you need to do something, you will figure out a way to do it.

Provide yourself a shorter amount of time to finish your work to eliminate diversions. It is like an artificial deadline to give yourself but backed up with something that holds you accountable. Tell your boss or client that you will provide them with a draft of a project by the end of the day. Find a partner for accountability that will hold you to your target time frame.

Setting a hard deadline; however, you do, and it will help you avoid distractions and amplify your productivity.

d.      Monitor your wandering mind.

According to one Harvard study, we spend almost 50 percent of our waking time thinking about something other than what we're supposed to be doing. We're on autopilot, and our mind wanders, partly to avoid trying to concentrate on something. The key to increased productivity is to notice when the mind is distracted and to bring the task back to your attention.

It implies paying attention to your thoughts and knowing when your mind begins to drift. It permits you to manage what you concentrate on when you mistake and to redirect your thoughts. You actively placed the brakes on this disturbance instead of allowing your own to keep meandering over to social networks to check out your information feed.

Pay attention to what distractions are challenging to prevent so that you can catch them sooner. Take a breath when you feel a desire to give in to a distraction and purposely choose not to respond to it. It's tougher to regroup and bring your focus back to the job at hand when you have given in and permitted yourself to focus on another thing, like reading e-mails.

2.    In short, instead of allowing yourself to skip between tasks and distractions, be mindful of your thoughts.

a.    By making a game out of it, train your brain.

3.    Like a muscle, your mind is. It would help if you built it up to use it effectively. By gradually working on our concentration, we need to train our brains to stay focused. It will reinforce our ability for more extended periods to focus.

4. An excellent means to begin doing this is through the "Pomodoro Technique, "in which you set a timer and, for an amount of time, 45 minutes straight, are entirely focused on a task. Then allow a 15-minute break for yourself.

5. Start with something more manageable, such as 25 minutes, if 45 minutes is a stretch, and then give yourself a five-minute break. The idea is to make it a game—to challenge yourself to work on your assignment diligently until the timer rings. Then allow yourself, but only for an allotted time, to gorge on whatever distraction you want.

6. It's back to working again after the break until the timer rings. You'll be amazed at how much using this method you can get done!

a. Take on more demanding work.

7. It may be that your work does not fully engage you if you have trouble concentrating and are chronically distracted. You may feel like

you're working hard all day, but your mind might be fighting boredom and looking for something more interesting to fill the time with.

8. Complex tasks require more of our memory and attention at work, which means that we have less mental capacity to wander to the nearest stimulating distraction. When our skills are challenged, we're most likely to enter a state of total work immersion. When our abilities greatly exceed our work requirements, we get bored—such as when we do mindless data entry for several hours.

9. Evaluate the level of unproductive busy work that you do. Are you having a hard time getting involved in the plan? It could suggest that you can take on more challenging projects. We can be consumed and hyper-focused on the job when we tackle a much more intricate job that presses our capacity and intellectual limits. Our minds are wired to concentrate on anything one-of-a-kind, positive or enormous. And

tackling these tasks provides us with a sense of accomplishment.

10.    With a task we deem menial, we have no such sense of accomplishment.

a.    Break your stress and distraction cycle.

11.    Stress can also play a significant part in our inability to concentrate or overcome distractions. Too often, while feeling overwhelmed, we find ourselves trying to work. It leaves us frazzled and exhausted, distracted easily, and unable to concentrate. It can suggest that you're under raised tension if you're conveniently distracted.

12.    "There's even a name for it: "anxiety that is easily distracted." Symptoms include:

13.    You have trouble concentrating, and your mind continually drifts away from what you focus on.

14.    You have more trouble forming ideas and staying on track than usual.

15.     Your thoughts feel muddled and impaired.

16.     Your short-term memory is not as good as it usually is, you feel.

17.     It will assist you in regaining your focus and overcoming distractions more efficiently by bringing your stress under control. To decrease the body's stress response, you must find ways to calm your mind and relax your body. Make sure there's enough sleep you get. Practice exercises for breathing and find ways to reduce your anxiety.

## Evaluation Question

1. What can I do to set my goal?

2. How can I benefit from my goal for me to achieve what I want?

3. Why do I need a goal?

## Note yourself Improvement in this chapter

_____

_____

_____

_____

_____

_____

_____

_____

_____

_____

_____

_____

_____

# TEN(10) STAGES TO FINDING THE POSITIVE IN ANY CIRCUMSTANCE

**<u>The most effective method to consistently look on the brilliant side of life:</u>** 10 stages to finding the positive in any circumstance

*"A few things in life are awful*

*They can truly make you frantic*

*Different things simply cause you to swear and revile.*

*At the point when you're biting on life's cartilage*

*Try not to protest, give a whistle*

*Furthermore, that'll help things show up for the .....BEST!*

Also, consistently look on the splendid side of life... (whistle along... )

Continuously look on the light side of life... " (by Eric Idle)

It is one of my main tunes EVER. I love the film The Life of Brian by the British Monty Python group, and this tune ALWAYS makes me grin; truth be told, I can't hear it without an expansive grin crossing my face, even in the most noticeably awful circumstances. That, and Bring Me Sunshine by Morecombe and Wise's and Take On Me by Aha. Alright, so those last two may be only exceptional to me. However, there's something so magnificent about music that blends the spirit and lifts our disposition that it merits helping ourselves remember exactly how incredible a few things can be. I wager you're singing this melody quietly in your mind now – it's appealing, and the words truly have tremendous importance – if you let them.

Yet, there's the rub – 'if you let them.' Many of us experience life are taking a gander at all the negative things in our day-to-day existence that we miss large numbers of the superb, positive, and insisting things that are around us constantly. In the law of fascination terms, that is simply going to bring us a greater amount of what we've centered around – the undesirable negative things.

So how would you generally look on the splendid side of life to draw in a greater amount of what you need? Here are ten quick and simple tips to help you.

## 1. Avoid adverse things and contrary individuals

It is a critical one for me and basic regarding the law of fascination, which expresses that 'where center goes, energy streams.' You will draw in negative energy on the off chance that you are continually around adverse individuals, which will deplete you quicker than water streaming out of a shower. We as a whole know the sort of individuals, I mean – the ones where nothing at any point goes appropriate for them, and they are distraught except if there is something to groan about. What they are neglecting to see is that terrible things happen to everybody eventually. What is significant isn't what occurs; however, how we manage what occurs. That is the thing that decides our results, not simply the occasions. You can't help individuals who have secured a twisting of negative deduction by being hauled somewhere around their 'stuff.' So if you need to put some distance between you and the negative musings of another, do it! That frequently implies killing the news, putting down the paper, and helping yourself to remember a decent story you as of late heard all things being equal. It doesn't mean disregarding a companion out of luck or choosing not to see. However, you will be greatly improved at aiding your companion or finding an answer for an issue if you are in a decent and positive spot yourself, instead of if you are both emptying the energy of the other like a clairvoyant vampire!

## 2. Locate the positive in each circumstance

There is one – every time! Yeah, there is one! And if you can't see it, it's because you don't look enough at the large image: like a fly that continues to float in glass. After all, it can't draw far enough to see that a window at the top is open! If your car breaks down, it could warn you that your attention is needed, and a more serious issue may save your life. If you break your leg or are sick, ask yourself what you're trying to prevent and whether it will lead you in a whole new direction if you have time to rest and focus on your life. Hopefully, you will build a bigger strategy from within that will lead you to your position in the end. Trust: a diversion in the street is often required to prevent falling into the water!

## 3. Think – take a full breath

Goodness indeed, indeed, yes. It is one of my top picks as well. Stop, take in gradually for eight, forgets about, and inhale gradually for eight checks. Presently rehash that until you have done it multiple times. Doesn't that vibe better? Breathing profoundly and expanding our oxygen admission can decrease pressure and strain, improve your insusceptible framework and detoxify your body. It is the most common cure on the planet, and we would all be able to improve by getting more engaged and mindful of the breath going through us. Figuring out how to clear your mind through reflection and breathing is probably the best thing you can do to change your mentality and improve your enthusiasm and actual well-being. There are numerous breathing methods like yoga, Tai chi, and Qigong, which can likewise profit your disposition if you study them.

## 4. Be thankful for the things you have – remember you're good fortune

How frequently have you said 'thank you today for the things you as of now have? Have you put your consideration on all the incredible things around you, or have you zeroed in additional on the absence of things you have? Do you have this in context? The way that you are perusing this on a P.C. or cell phone implies that you will, in any event, approach a specific level of abundance that is more than the vast majority on the planet have. However, you approach power did you realize that almost 25 percent of the number of inhabitants in all non-industrial nations had no power in a new report – which means over 1.3 billion individuals were living in obscurity. One in nine individuals on the planet doesn't approach clean water near and dear. How do your issues look now? <u>There is an incredible Ralph McTell tune called The Streets of London which says:</u>

*"How could you say to me that you are lonely and say that the sun does not shine for you?*

*Let me grab your hand and guide you through the streets of London,*

I'm going to show you things that will make you change your mind."

So check out you today and be appreciative of the things you have now have – that is a guaranteed approach to get a greater amount of the things you love. Zeroing in on need brings more need. Say 'thank you for your favors and watch a greater amount of the stream into your life.

## 5. Utilize your enthusiastic knowledge to comprehend what is truly occurring in a circumstance – separate current realities from your feelings

We, as a whole, every so often, let our feelings improve us. Without a doubt, I would contend that tuning in to your feelings is essential as we should know about how we are feeling and why to change things. In any case, allowing your feelings to control your life isn't prudent since we regularly settle on more unfortunate decisions and make sketchy moves when we are in the hold of low recurrence feelings like scorn, outrage, dread, or desire. Having the option to disassociate yourself from the circumstance by venturing back and taking a gander at it in a more targeted way is vital. Having passionate insight is fundamental. That isn't equivalent to saying you ought never to feel furious (or other such feelings). I blow up now and then, we as a whole do, yet I attempt to perceive that I am permitting myself to blow up, make a full breath and stride back from the circumstance and my negative feelings. I frequently ask myself, "if I was a fly on the divider here as opposed to being sincerely included, what might my point of view be at that point?" When I do that, I understand that the individual who cut me up in the vehicle in front is truly much the same as me, behind schedule for work and focused on it. At that point, I can decide to release my annoyance and separate my feelings from current realities. Also, when I do that, I, for the most part, locate that the vehicle ahead turns off at any rate, and I'm back to where I began.

## 6. Accomplish something physical

There is a lot of information supporting how doing some actual exercise helps your body truly. But there is also a lot of proof that exercise will benefit you mentally, too. It can diminish mellow to direct melancholy by delivering common endorphins and different synapses in mind like serotonin, which can lift your mindset. Exercise likewise diminishes pressure and can lessen strain in the body, giving you more energy, improved rest, and a superior capacity to confront life's difficulties. It doesn't matter what sort of activity you do, yet standard measures of activity can help you look on the splendid side of life because of these impacts. You can begin with 5 minutes per day or 10-15 minutes each 2-3 days. All that you do will assist with your psychological just as your actual well-being.

Furthermore, it's hard to feel hopeless when hopping around your family room to your main tune, so get up and move it! Another approach to help is through tapping. I've composed a post about tapping (otherwise called the enthusiastic opportunity strategy), which can effectively affect your passion and actual well-being by delivering blocks in the body's energy frameworks. It's a simple and free approach to life your temperament with the goal that you can value the positive in any circumstance. Peruse more about tapping here.

## 7. Play a portion of your #1 music

It is a truly straightforward and successful strategy for lifting your state of mind – recollect the beginning of this post. The explanation that music functions admirably is that it tends to be an 'anchor' for an inclination or positive feeling. If you feel a forceful feeling when you hear, see, contact or smell something, an association is made in the cerebrum between the 'thing' you heard, saw, contacted, or tasted and the disposition or state you were in. When you later experience that thing once more, your cerebrum consequently returns you to the first passionate state. So if you felt exceptionally upbeat when you initially heard a specific tune, and it helps you to remember a glad time in your life, when you hear it once more, your body returns you to a cheerful state. Securing is an NLP procedure that you can use to lift your state of mind whenever. I will compose a post on mooring soon as it merits something beyond a couple of words here. Nonetheless, for the motivations behind this rundown, consider putting on your number one music or taking a gander at a most loved picture can assist put you with support a positive, passionate state.

## 8. Compose a rundown, mull over it, at that point, read it back

Recording things can assist with getting sorted out your contemplations. Giving yourself a couple of hours away and afterward perusing things back will permit you some distance between your underlying responses to an occasion and a more target perspective. If you are battling to locate a splendid side to a specific circumstance, get a piece of paper and compose two headings: positive and negative. On the negative side, record your sentiments about the circumstance in negative terms. You might have the option to do this openly since it is the state you are in at that specific second.

On the contrary, side, think about certain things that you can and record these as well. Ask yourself, 'what openings do I presently have that I didn't see previously?' You might be shocked at the appropriate responses. For instance, breaking your arm may appear to be something terrible at that point; however, on the off chance that you ask yourself what openings you currently have. You could concoct some sure things like more opportunity to rest and unwind, more opportunity to explore a vocation change you generally needed, a chance to review the equilibrium of tasks in your family. For instance, if you have been the just one doing all the errands, breaking your arm could help you rebalance the responsibility. Making a rundown like this can truly assist you with seeing things from an alternate perspective. Give yourself some time before you read back. The fundamental considerations often help detach you from the underlying emotions, and you might find that the 'bad' rundown may seem to be an over-response when you read it back.

## 9. Chuckle and snicker once more

Giggling discharges endorphins in the mind which are the body's characteristic feel-acceptable synthetic substances. Snickering can reduce pressure and increment your safe cells and contamination, battling antibodies that can protect your infection. At times the lone activity in a negative circumstance is to see its entertaining side. Step back from the pressure and chuckle. I frequently utilize this with my youngsters when something they do turns out badly and promptly understand their error. Rather than yelling, I attempt to snicker, which diffuses their feelings and stress, and they wind up giggling as well. When they were 7 and 9, they inquired whether they could evaluate some face paints higher up. I said indeed, and everything went calm. Around 20 minutes after the fact, the two young ladies came bobbing into the room, totally exposed however painted from head to toe in various examples and tones – and I mean from head to toe! They were both so satisfied with themselves that I was unable to discover it in my heart to be furious. We snickered, all things being equal – I lauded them for their cunning innovativeness and creative examples, and we chuckled and giggled some more. What's more, wiping off the hand and impressions from the dividers and rails in the house was truly not unreasonably troublesome!

## 10. Reexamine the circumstance

It is a key NLP strategy to help you see the positives. It essentially implies taking a gander at the circumstance diversely and putting an alternate 'outline' around it. Frequently you see things contrarily because you have put a specific 'outline' around the circumstance, and you can't see outside it. For instance, if you have started to want to wed your accomplice and they cut off your association, you may end up not being able to see anything outside of the casing you made about being hitched to that individual. You will be unable to review that you contended a great deal and that you didn't have similar convictions and qualities. Reexamining the circumstance will permit you to put an alternate casing around it. If you ask yourself what outline your companion may put on the circumstance or your mum, you may then see reality regarding how frequently you contended all things considered. Thus, that could lead you to find in the circumstance differently, and you might be eased that you had a lucky break from being hitched to an individual with whom you regularly oppose this idea. **I've recorded some other normal rethinks underneath, too; however, truly; these will be however individual as you seem to be:**

- **Lost your job** - consider this to be a chance to go into business or as an approach to change your profession when maybe you were frightened to try and consider the big picture previously

- **<u>Divorced or unloaded</u>** – again, this could be a chance to escape a broken relationship or address things that were not working in the relationship yet, you were disregarding for reasons unknown or another

- **<u>Failing</u>** – on the off chance that you can reevaluate 'disappointment' as accomplishing an alternate result from the one you at first needed, you will go far in finding the splendid side of life. It's tied in with seeing the improvement you have made instead of zeroing in on the one thing you haven't: Imagine you are shooting a bolt at an objective. You hit eight rather than ten and might suspect you have fizzled. Rethinking this implies advising yourself that you shot the bolt in any case, hit the objective, and got 80% of the aggregate. Accomplishing the following 20% is currently just a basic advance of changing the point instead of discarding everything and beginning once more.

- **<u>No cash</u>** – there will consistently be individuals with more and short of what you. There will be individuals who are taller, more limited, fatter, more slender! Continually zeroing in on the absence of things in your day-to-day existence, be it cash, love, well-being, or whatever else, will bring you business as usual because the law of fascination will coordinate your sentiments with business usual. To reevaluate the present circumstance, start by appreciating what you do have – there will be parcels to celebrate. If you need some motivation, recall that numerous individuals in history have returned from the verge monetarily. Walt Disney couldn't take care of his bills in his initial vocation, and his first organization failed after a wholesaler created them. However, that didn't stop him, and in 1928, he dispatched the initially vivified film with audio effects entitled Steamboat Willie, acquainting the world with Mickey Mouse - the rest is history.

Furthermore, if that is sufficiently not - what about Abraham Lincoln, Henry Ford, and H. J. Heinz (of the 57 assortments distinction). Every one of them failed before finding monetary achievement. Seemingly the finish to them was truly the start.

- **<u>Dark Night of the spirit</u>** - this could be viewed as the absolute bottom in someone's life. Furthermore, it is a troublesome, however generally essential, occasion for the individual to learn something important to them in otherworldliness terms. At times the reevaluation is to acknowledge that there is nothing to do except for giving up. Esther Hicks allegorically says that if you leap out of the plane without a parachute, now and again, the lone activity is to understand that it will all be over soon. Numerous individuals need to arrive in a desperate predicament to understand their latent capacity and bob back. One of the best account structures in movies, books, and books includes the 'legend's excursion' where the saint consistently faces their 'dim evening of the spirit.' The least snapshot of their life, not long before they find their actual force and proceed to defeat their adversary. So if you are confronting a dim evening of the spirit in your own life, burrow profound inside yourself and discover your flexibility. Put stock in yourself, and you will discover the solidarity to proceed. I don't accept that the universe brings you anything you can't survive. However, you may need to pose yourself some awkward inquiries and do some spirit looking through first.

## DETERMINATION AND SUCCESS

### <u>How vital are determination and drive for success?</u>
The drive is a typical quality among successful people.

The bright side is that just like luck and success, the drive is a continuum. There are instances where individuals with marginal drive enjoy what they do and experience huge success. On the other end of the range, you find ruthless fixation.

**<u>What happens if you aren't normally driven?</u>** Here once again, there's excellent information. You can embrace successful methods. What you lack in character, you can offset in strategy.

Right here are refreshing take away:

i. The drive is the one common feature among effective individuals. The one point all successful people share is drive and also a decision.

ii. The drive ranges from enjoyment to fierce fixation. Drive can go from simply delighting in the path to what individuals would consider "a little mad," implying a callous fascination for results.

iii. A need for personal power. One reason for drive is a search for personal power or an extension of character.

iv. A suggestion shackles them. Some individuals come to be taken in by a concept. Their drive is sustained by the passion for bringing an idea to life.

v. The decision to end up the task: some people are fueled by an interest in completing what they started. They cannot stand the idea of leaving something half-finished.

vi. You don't have to transform your character. If you're not normally driven, you don't need to try to change your individuality. Instead, adopt tested success methods that define effective people.

vii. Adopt success strategies of effective people. You can embrace tested techniques such as coming to be a lot more single-minded and concentrated, a strong orientation, don't take no for a response, and become better at saying what you don't, such as.

What I've learned with experience is that you require to know what you're trading while the drive is necessary. For example, look for a balance between your sentence and your connection, so you do not melt bridges or leave a corps route in your search of results. Attempt to get your body connections and enjoyment throughout the pursuit of your objectives as you delight in the process. Goals are a car; they are a method to an end; however, not the end themselves. Be careful not to endanger your worth along your journey.

## Drive is the one usual characteristic of successful individuals

### *Determination is the one typical characteristic amongst successful individuals:*

"As the readers will certainly uncover in this publication, effective people are usually really single-minded and determined. Without a doubt, it would certainly be feasible to select this out as the one particularly common to mostly all effective people. It might take the form of a drive: if you want something hard enough, you will obtain it. It can take the kind of brutality: allow absolutely nothing to stand between you and your goal. It can take the form of a solid sense of objective. It can take the type of resolution and determination: approve failing only as an action on the path to success."

### ✓ *One Single Goal*

"This sort of resolution resembles fanaticism and also what may be called 'a little madness'. It implies a rather strange sight of life because one single goal becomes more important than any others. A person might agree to compromise his wife, children, pals, health and wellness, and even his life for this goal. Sometimes the goal might appear quite like a fascination. At its extreme, desire is a kind of insanity."

### ✓ *An Orientation Urges Action*

"There are lots of advantages to an effective determination as well as a strong orientation. The sense of direction urges action. The orientation shapes the activity. The sense of direction allows the worth of the activity to be examined: has it got me nearer to my goal? The orientation permits all judgments and decisions to be made more conveniently: does this help me towards my objective, or does this prevent me? Most people in their normal lives lack such a strong feeling of worth when making a choice. Many people may need to consider a soup of different elements such as family, wellness, satisfaction, profession, etc., when choosing. The strongly-success-oriented individual thinks about something: the course to success."

✓ *Determination Ranges from Satisfaction to Fascination*

"As with good luck, there is, obviously, a range. At one end is the ruthless obsessed autocrat that can effectively be called mad. At the various other ends of the spectrum is the person who appreciates what they are doing, enjoys his life and friends, and seems to stumble into success (as with Nolan Bushnell, Norman Lear, or Sir Clive Sinclair). Readers may be amazed to locate that most of the people in this publication appear to fall under this second grouping."

### ✓ *Adopt Techniques to Improve Efficiency*

"A person that will certainly not take 'no' for an answer and also composes ten letters runs the threat of being a problem, and a bug, however, might be more effective than the individual who is turned off by first rejection. Such things may develop normally from individuality, or they may be taken on as a method. You cannot will certainly on your own have a nasty temper (also if this typically seems to be most valuable for success). However, you can come to be much better at stating what you do not like. It may well be that having success-oriented features under your character is far more reliable-- nonetheless adopting some of them as calculated approaches can likewise be valuable."

## Purpose And Enthusiasm

"Where there's a will, there's away. If there's a million possibility that you can do anything, something, to prevent what you want from stopping, do it. Tear the door open or, if demand is, wedge your foot because the door and also maintain it open."-- Pauline Kael

The background has revealed some individuals conquered overwhelming odds to be successful. For example, many successful entrepreneurs have been diagnosed with a developmental reading disorder, like dyslexia, including popular Virgin Richard Branson. Daniel Pink, the writer of An Entire New Mind, points out Sally Shaywitz, a Yale neuroscientist and dyslexia specialist who says: "Dyslexics think differently. They are instinctive as well as excel at analytic, seeing the huge image as well as streamlining. They are poor rote reciters but motivated dreamers." People with dyslexia have to get over huge odds to succeed, which indicates a solid will to thrive. It is estimated that several top international Chief

Executive Officer's past and existing are dyslexic. How about you? What have you got over in your life?

The human will is, without a doubt, powerful. Once a strict commitment is made to perform a task or objective, there's little to quit for an individual. You might have heard it stated that the human will could relocate any hill. As long as one's will certainly is undaunted and sustained with the appropriate objectives, individuals can conquer most challenges on their roadway to success. Perseverance comes to be the guy's greatest ally for success. Will and also goal come to be powerful factors required to realize one's objective. The various other essential feature is objective as well as interest. An objective is defined as recognizing our role within the structure of life. It is the capacity to harness our skills, talents, and wizard with a direct, focused focus on a quest. A deliberate vision is an extension of these professors since it coincides with a common goal that benefits humankind. We might conclude that combining a strong will with objective creates a deliberate vision clothed with honorable intentions. Lots of pioneers have accomplished huge success even with dominating external circumstances. As an example, Albert Einstein once specified: "Great spirits have always come across terrible opposition from mediocre minds."

# Habits of people with remarkable determination

How effective individuals stand up to lure, stay concentrated, identified, and continue to be undaunted in search of their goals.

Doing all you need to do to be successful, with complete focus and resolve, is incredibly difficult.

It is why the ability to work hard and react positively to failure and difficulty is important. Resolve, self-control, and determination help successful individuals work hard and stick to their lasting objectives.

Right here are ways you can establish those high qualities also-- and because of this be a lot more successful:

a. Let your past inform your future-- and nothing even more.

- The past is valuable. Pick up from your mistakes. Learn from the mistakes of others.

- Then let it go.

- Easier said than done? It relies on your viewpoint. When something poor occurs to you, see it as a possibility to learn something you didn't understand. When one more individual makes a mistake, don't just learn from it-- see it as an opportunity to be kind, forgiving, as well as compassionate.

- The past is just preparation; it doesn't describe you. Consider what failed, but only in terms of how you will see to it that next time, you as well as the people around you will recognize exactly how to make sure it goes right.

b.    **See your life– and future– as entirely within your control.**

There's a quote typically credited to Ignatius: "Hope as if God will care for all; act as if all is up to you."The very same premise applies to luck. Lots of people feel good luck has a whole lot to do with success or failure. If they prosper, good luck preferred them, and also, if they fall short, good fortune was against them.

The majority of successful people do feel good luck played some function in their success. Yet they don't wait at all the best or bother with bad luck. They behave as if success or failure is completely within their control. If they prosper, they caused it. If they fall short, they caused it.

By not losing mental energy, worrying about what may happen to you, you can place all your initiative right into making things occur. (And then, if you obtain, fortunately, hello, you're even better off.).

You can't control luck. However, you can control yourself.

c. **Learn to ignore the important things you can have no control over.**

Mental stamina resembles muscular tissue toughness-- nobody has a limitless supply. So why drain your strength on something that you can't control?

For some individuals, it's politics; for others, it's household; it's global warming among some. Whatever it is, you care for it, and you want someone to take care of it. Okay, do what you can do: Ballot. Lend a paying attention ear. Reuse, and also reduce your carbon impact. Do what you can do. Be your change-- but don't attempt to make every person else change.

d. **Don't resent, however, rather commemorate the success of others.**

Many people-- I ensure you know at least a few-- see success as a zero-sum game: There's just a lot to go around. When another person radiates, they think that diminishes the light from their stars.

Resentment sucks up a substantial amount of mental power-- power much better applied somewhere else.

When a pal does something awesome, that doesn't preclude you from doing something outstanding. Where success is concerned, birds of a plume tend to flock with each other-- so attract your effective buddies also more detailed.

Don't dislike awesomeness. Develop and celebrate awesomeness anywhere you discover it, and in time you'll find even more of it in yourself.

e. **Never stoop to complaining, slamming, or worrying.**

Your words have control, particularly over you; worrying about your problems only makes you feel worse, not better. So if something is incorrect, don't waste time grumbling. Put that mental energy right into making the situation better. (Unless you intend to whine concerning it for life, at some point, you'll have to make it much better.).

So why lose time? Repair it currently. Don't talk about what's incorrect. Speak about how you'll make things better; also, if that discussion is only with yourself.

f. **Constantly review your lasting goals.**

Claim you intend to construct a bigger business; when you're emotionally worn out, it's very easy to justify doing much less than your best. Say you intend to slim down; when you're emotionally worn out, it's very easy to rationalize that you'll begin changing your consuming as well as workout practices tomorrow. Say you intend to engage better with the employees; when you're psychologically tired, it's easy to reason that you truly need to work on that report instead.

Psychological exhaustion makes us take the very easy escape-- even though the easy way takes us the wrong way.

The key is to produce concrete suggestions that draw you back from the impulse brink. A pal has a duplicate of his bank note taped to his computer system screen as a continuous reminder of a commitment he must satisfy. One more maintains a photo of himself on his refrigerator taken when he weighed 50 pounds a lot more to work as a consistent tip of the individual he never wishes to be once more. Another loads his desk with family pictures, both since he enjoys considering them and advising himself of individuals he is ultimately benefiting.

Consider minutes when you are most likely to give in to impulses that take you further away from your long-term objectives. Then use concrete suggestions of those long-term goals to interrupt the motivation and keep you on track.

Or better yet, revamp your setting so you eliminate your ability to be spontaneous. Then you don't need to work out any type of willpower whatsoever. If you can state no to examining your social media site accounts every couple of minutes, transform them off as well as put them away for several hours each time, so you don't have to be solid enough to say no.

1. What should be done to be determined?

2. Who do I make friends with so I can be determined?

3. What should be done to prevent me from complaining?

4. How can my lasting goal be reviewed?

5. What can be done to avoid the past from affecting my future?

**Note yourself Improvement in this chapter**

_____

_____

_____

_____

---------------------------------------

---------------------------------------

---------------------------------------

---------------------------------------

---------------------------------------

---------------------------------------

---------------------------------------

---------------------------------------

---------------------------------------

---------------------------------------

## FORMING HABITS OF SUCCESS

**How long can a new habit take to be established?**
The time duration can range from a solitary second to
some years. The speed of new behavior pattern
growth is significantly figured out by the strength of
the emotion that goes along with choosing to start
acting in a specific way.

Many people assume, speak about, and resolve to
reduce weight as well as become healthy. This talk

might go on for years. Then someday, the medical professional states, "If you don't get your weight down and also enhance your physical condition, you remain at threat of passing away at an early age."

All of a sudden, the thought of passing away can be so extreme or frightening that the specific promptly changes his diet plan, starts working out, quits cigarette smoking, and also comes to be a healthy and balanced and fit person. Psychotherapists describe this as a "significant emotional experience" or a "SEE." Any experience of extreme delight or pain incorporated with behavior can trigger a new action pattern that may endure for the remainder of an individual's life.

For example, setting your hand on a hot oven or touching a live electric wire will give you an intense as well as immediate discomfort or shock. The experience might only take a fraction of a second. For the rest of your life, though, you'll possess the behavior of not putting your hand on a hot oven or touching live electric cords. The habits will undoubtedly have been created immediately as well as will sustain ultimately.

According to the professionals, it takes about 21 days to develop a habit pattern of tool intricacy. By this, we indicate basic behaviors such as getting up early, exercising each morning before you start, listening to audio programs in your automobile, going to bed at a particular hour, being punctual for consultations, planning daily beforehand, and beginning with your most essential jobs daily or completing one task before you start something else. These are behaviors of medium complexity that can be relatively quickly developed over three weeks with technique and rep.

**Exactly how do you establish a new behavior?** Over the years, a straightforward, powerful, proven approach has been developed for new habit development. It's quite like a recipe for preparing a dish in the kitchen-- you can use it to acquire any practice you want. With time, you'll discover it much more comfortable and also less complicated to create the behaviors you wish to incorporate right into your personality.

Most of us can recognize that good habits are much better than bad habits, yet there is still a clear gap between intention-to-action and action.

New habits development techniques focus on setup, context, obstacles to action, social impact, and emotion. Still, these should be unpacked on an instance-by-case basis and do not frequently provide an extensive spread method that many people can use.

Nonetheless, our understanding of how we proactively create new habits in the brain has helped develop new behavior and habits that last. To understand these, we initially need to comprehend the dynamics of a habit.

# The science behind habits

A habit is a spontaneous behavioral pattern in feedback to a hint. It's the result of duplicating a behavior in the very same context again and again. It occurs when we distort up our seat belts when we get in a vehicle, dive onto Facebook when we are feeling burnt out, or bear in mind to take a notepad with us to a meeting.

Repetition enhances the link in the brain between a hint and the associated behavior. With enough repetition, our actions relocate from being initially mindful practices to subconscious practice.

The key is that repetition is vital. Exactly how we relocate from new behavior to practice can be likened to learning to drive a car and truck. When we operate for the first time, we felt too aware of what we were doing and continuously remembered putting the gear stick into 2nd gear when we moved with a corner. Yet, gradually and with repetition, we can't also purposely keep shifting equipment after being driven somewhere on the same day.

The brain enjoys hardwiring thinking, yet it has little ability to do this. We can only excel in improving one habit at a time. It is why we can talk on the phone and drive as soon as we've mastered driving a car (assuming you're using a hands-free tool), yet not when we were initially learning to do so.

## Small actions, big rewards

Usually, we anticipate considerable modifications in our behavior and set challenging objectives: Shed 38kgs, awaken at 5 am, make $10 million in the first year of business. The fact is that change and the formation of new practices are tiny and calls for incremental repetitive steps to take hold.

When we have a soaring objective, we commonly get discouraged when we don't see substantial progress. It restricts our desire to duplicate the behavior that is called for by the mind to produce new habits. So, what's the option?

We require to piece our objectives into smaller behaviors that can be accomplished conveniently as well as always. When we attain a goal, the brain releases dopamine, the feel-good hormonal agent, and adrenaline, the power hormone. It develops an upward spiral where we feel determined and also have the energy to achieve much more.

So, rather than functioning towards a $10 million target, break down that goal into a piece of lead-generating task a day. This success of smaller incremental goals will produce a harmony of dopamine and adrenaline in the mind associated with the behavior that will allow us to ride this wave in a positive higher spiral of rep in time.

## I-Then plan and how to use them

Behavioral researchers recommend that we create a regular that weaves our new preferred behavior into our everyday lives to enhance repetition to become a default action and a habit eventually. It calls for regularity, a reminder to do so, and most notably, what some researchers call an If-Then plan.

It is a cue in our mind to behave in a particular means when a scenario presents itself. It is aided by stacking brand-new preferred practices into existing behaviors. As an example, we can develop an If-Then strategy to head to the health club after functioning by ensuring that once we get home after work and also obtain changes out of our work clothing (If), we obtain clothed into our fitness center clothing (Then).

It creates an achievable and easily repeatable behavior (getting ready for fitness center) that enables us to develop a positive higher spiral (launching dopamine and adrenaline) to satisfy a bigger, more crucial objective (boosted total health and wellness).

As soon as we can produce this loose link in mind between wanted task(Then) and situational cue (If), this connected behavior becomes quickly obtainable in mind and, therefore, less complicated to remember. Once we have recalled it enough, it is hardwired and comes to be a new routine, relocating from the aware to the subconscious.

---

### Drawing it all with each other

What objectives are you currently working with to bring down into smaller-sized goals to produce a positive upward spiral? How can you develop If-Then strategies or psychological signs to see if your wanted practices are simple to recall and act on based on adding your day-to-day environment? However, beginning small, that's how you form the behaviors that will inevitably lead you down a path of success.

### Breaking the habits holding you back from success

Bad habits are part of being human; if they're bad enough, they can take control of you and also steer your life in incorrect directions. Bad habits can be unfavorable self-talk, disadvantageous behaviors, or outright self-devastating vices like medicines and cigarettes. Lots of people have tried to stop their low actions yet have had restricted success. They relapsed back into the old practice and placed it into the 'too hard basket' to think of a few other times.

Breaking your bad habits implies re-shaping your neurology; your brain is designed to seek enjoyment and also avoid discomfort. If your poor behavior provides you short-term (perceived) pleasure and even giving up gives you pain, you can find yourself in a bind. If your mind acquires more satisfaction than discomfort from an act, it will seek enjoyment. When the behavior develops more pain than pleasure, you'll begin moving away from it. You'll duplicate the very same actions unless you re-wire your brain for a different result.

Altering the habit takes time and repetition, don't expect to change the routine you've already had for years overnight. The decision can be reached in a second. But the new practice requires time to embed itself into your subconscious. Your new patterns of behavior need to override the old. Destructive behaviors should be replaced by more productive as well as empowering ones.

Here are some strategies that can assist you to transform the habits and also change your life:

### Do i revise my self-image?

Your self-image controls your thoughts, activities, and your whole life; your practices develop around what you think yourself to be. For example, take the procrastination habit; if you hesitate, you may begin recognizing it as a slow starter'. Individuals' behavior mirrors how they see themselves. Labeling yourself as a procrastinator is like offering your authorization to hesitate; each time you postpone, your identification is reinforced, and an adverse comments loophole is formed.

The opposite is also true; if you identify yourself as a success and reaffirm your capability to obtain points done, you solidify your self-identification as an effective individual. Your thoughts and activities are then straightened with the identification of a successful individual.

## How to start revising your self-image?

So how do you begin to change your self-image?

- Begin with a clear idea of who you wish to be and also what you intend to have.

- Choose what practices and habits you intend to embed right into your individuality.

- Visualize on your own doing those new practices.

- See yourself in your mind's eye as the individual you want to be.

- Visualize your living the life you want to have.

- Re-shape your neurology. Neurons that terminate together a cable with each other.

- Take advantage of the mind's strength to become who you want to be; the human mind is plastic; you can essentially alter your brain.

- The modification is a subtle and steady procedure; you won't see the adjustment up until it's currently happened.

- Modify your self-image by seeing yourself as somebody new.

- Start doing new behaviors that are straightened with the individual you intend to be.

- Set new goals as well as review books.

- Bombard your mind with stimulation about your brand-new self-image.

## Focus on little success

Don't establish your bar so high that your mind won't believe you can do it. When you want to change a negative behavior, don't expect that you have to stand up to the routine every day for the rest of your life; begin with one day, one week, then one month. If a behavior has been developed and repeated over the years, don't stress yourself to transform overnight. Set up little wins for yourself, then stack them on top of each other; this way, you get momentum and confidence, making the more significant objectives come easier; bringing a big goal right into smaller pieces makes it much more workable. Make long-term progression one small win at once.

## Complacency is your enemy

Complacency is the enemy of success, and idleness and complacency eliminate your initiatives to damage negative habits by destroying any kind of energy you've built up. Get comfortable being uncomfortable; once you have transformed your behavior and stopped a practice, you still require to be attentive not to relapse right into the old behavior;

repeating that ancient practice even once will take you back to the start. Your unwelcome neural bond is still intact; if you reawaken it, you'll be right back to where you began.

Recuperating alcoholics and addicts can be sober for many years, yet they understand that they'll end up being an addict once more if they also take one drink or hit. Your harmful routines come back to haunt you if you let your guard down, remain cautious, and avoid complacency.

## Why should I change my old habit with a new one?

To effectively damage a harmful practice, you have to replace it with a much better one; your mind needs to concentrate on something new.

Have your mind active in a new behavior until it replaces the old routine and select a unique practice that makes your life much better and offers you pleasure and happiness. Reiterate and condition that habit into your life and be a new and much better you.

You can use this with all your negative behaviors, yet it's much easier to pick individually.

## Consider the long-term discomfort of your bad habits

You make the bad habit because, to a degree, it gives you gratification; if there were no enjoyment in the task, you wouldn't do it. Your behavior revolves around the pain/pleasure concept; this is why many people struck rock bottom before they do a total turn around and transform their lives. Think of the pleasure you get from your poor practice, then think of the long-term discomfort you will experience if you don't change it.

Use pain/pleasure to align your habits with what you want to be and what you want to have. Make a great life on your own. In some cases, just a few tiny modifications can make a tremendous difference

1.  How can I evaluate myself?

2. How do I become successful?

3. What is the bad habit that I need to change?

4. Which way do I deviate to become a successful being?

5. How do I focus on my little success?

6. How must I revise my self-image?

## Note yourself Improvement in this chapter

---------------------------------------------------------------
---------------------------------------------------------------
---------------------------------------------------------------
---------------------------------------------------------------
---------------------------------------------------------------
---------------------------------------------------------------
---------------------------------------------------------------
---------------------------------------------------------------
---------------------------------------------------------------
---------------------------------------------------------------
---------------------------------------------------------------
---------------------------------------------------------------
---------------------------------------------------------------
---------------------------------------------------------------

## THE HABIT OF MANAGING RESOURCES

Resources are things acquired for future use. When resources are not managed or maintained, it affects an individual in a long way.

Managers have had difficulty managing human resources are things for future use that are acquired. It affects an individual in a long way when resources are not managed or maintained resources for three reasons:

i. Cooperation, energy, and dedication from many employees are challenging to achieve in-depth, so managers are often unrealistic.

ii. Management concepts for large numbers of people often convey conflicting messages to managers.

iii. Some management assumptions regarding **HRM** undermine many managers' efforts, regardless of how well they are intended.

## Do I maintain my resources and how do I?

### Look for great lawful recommendations.

Good legal advice is crucial for your wealth to be preserved. Facing it, you can become a target when you get it to the top, and so you must protect your assets from predators. Lawyers should also check all business contracts, including those of their family and friends. Then if there's a dispute, ask the lawyer for advice before saying or doing one thing you may regret.

Keep up with what works for you – don't pursue the next hot investment.

The problem with the recent trends in money making is that they have no record - no success to look back on. Moreover, too many people seeking the same opportunities tend to benefit from new trends.

## Ensure yourself

Probably this is one of the biggest tips. Many companies are under-insured or are not insured against unavoidable disasters such as hurricanes, high winds, rain, floods, etc. Make sure you have an experienced, reputable insurance broker who can customize your insurance policies and investments.

## Immobilien investment.

Immobilien was the foundation of a tremendous fortune. If you want your real estate license to live financially free, learn and become an agent and investor, even though you will not be selling or transacting, you will understand what it means to invest in immovable.

Regardless of how you make money, real estate is the best way to preserve it because it is inflation-resistant if you invest long-term. There are likewise various tax advantages with the reality, which your Certified Public Accountant can usefully.

What I like about real estate, too, is that you don't have to sit asleep. If a stock or mutual fund moves up or up, your stock market investment can only show you a profit when you sell it other than if you have a small dividend due regularly. Your profits are up until then, a paper profit and still not a profit. But real estate can make money for you by leasing it and collecting rents while you own it.

It's all about keeping your money safe. That can sometimes mean to minimize taxation, to take precautions on those who want to make a piece of their money through litigation, to keep your principle up, and if possible, to take advantage of it. The aim of money protection, so that they can retire and then they can transfers, even their grandchildren.


The management challenge includes different methodologies employed by other teams, including milestones, iterative and collaborative methodologies. All benefit from a suitable type of work, but each has its difficulties that complicate resource management.

By combining different methodologies across various organizational maturities, companies are not uniquely responding to these challenges.

The benefits of management of business resources

Of course, we recognize that resource management is a complex process, particularly in a firm with shared, geographically scattered resources. With so many approaches, it should be meaningful that approaches to resource management can also change. **Each resource management software should include three capabilities, however:**

    i.    <u>Management of capacities and demand:</u> To optimize the use of resources by priority high-value work with available resources

    ii.    <u>Use of resources:</u> Ensure the right resources to support your strategic objectives

iii. <u>Advancements and Time Tracking:</u> Make sure you can track the progress of a particular value when using Time Tracking. Compare the planned effort to improve estimates and understand more precisely where your resources spend their time.

**<u>Using an effective corporate resource management system that provides these three skills, your company can:</u>**

A realistic view of both demand and the ability to deliver

i. Manage, prioritize, and establish adequate expectations with key stakeholders;

ii. Identify the availability of real resources

iii. Place the right resources at the right time for the right work

iv. Understand what roles and skills are required to meet commitments made by stakeholders

Increase and strengthen the partnership between project and research professionals and project partners

    i.     Finding problems earlier

    ii.    Provide objective work prioritization methods, ensuring a balance between demand and ability to deliver

    iii.   Connect implementation strategy

    iv.   Deliver innovation and transformation-friendly programs

## Engagement Of Employees

It is tough to capture the loyalty of hundreds or thousands of people in a business enterprise to direct their energies to the company's objectives. The company's objectives are long-term and general — profit and growth. However, employees usually concentrate on short periods to meet their wages, pay, working conditions, equitable treatment, and promotion needs. It is not easy to establish a relationship between these objectives.

## Relationships with people.

Group conduct theories address social interaction and interpersonal relationships using X and Y theories and sensitivity education.

Personal psychology, leadership, power, authority, responsibility, and subconscious is at the center of the individual behavior school of human relations.

Organizational development continues and concentrates on the need for people to discuss their daily difficulties together. Her central belief is that employees are often better able to manage themselves than managers can.

## Relations with the workforce.

Labor relations cover employment legislation, public policy, wage and cost economies, demographics, human resources management, collective bargaining, contracts management, and grievances. It views politics and employment law at the plant, corporate, union, state, and national level as the key to any situation. Her position is often adversarial and tough — she adheres to contractual conditions, refuses exemptions, avoids precedents, and creates a strong negotiating position.

Management of staff. The Province of Personnel is responsible for managing many people - namely the recruitment, selection, training, compensation, and development. This discipline states that companies will acquire employees with appropriate motives, habits, and conduct when performing these tasks well. Personnel maintains that a good climate will result when managers are consistent and apply policies that induce desired behavior.

Each school focuses on the development, but in very different ways of an influential, loyal, committed group of employees. It is not my concern that these experts are in disagreement or that the problem is addressed in different ways. I do not believe one school is right, the others are wrong, one school is better than another, or anyone should be ignored. They all supply suggestions and tools, which are usually incredibly helpful yet might not be used simultaneously.

## How to better deal with your money?

1.   **Hold a budget:** Many people don't budget for what they think will be a tedious process of listing expenditure, adding numbers, and ensuring that everything is aligned. You have no room for excuses with budgets if you're wrong with money. If it's all necessary for a

couple of hours of work that week to get your expenditure on track, why don't you make it here? Concentrate on the value that budgeting brings to your life rather than focus on creating the budget.

2.      **Budget:** if you make it and collect dust in a folder tucked away in your bookshelf or file office, your budget is useless. See it often throughout the month to guide your decisions about your spending. Upgrade it while you make compensation for fees and spend it on other monthly costs. You should always know how much money you can spend at any given time during the month, taking into account any expenses you have left to pay.

3.      **Give yourself an expenditure limit:** the net income or sum of money that is still available after you withdraw your costs from your income is a vital part of your budget. You can use the money for fun and entertainment, but only to a certain amount if you have any

money left over. With this money, you can't go crazy, especially if it's not a lot and lasts the whole month. Make sure you don't interfere with anything else you planned before making any massive purchases.

4.    **<u>Track your expenses here and there, small purchases add up quickly, and you have spent your budget before you know.</u>** Start monitoring your spending and identify regions where you may be uncertain. Save your receipts and write your purchases into an expenditure journal, categorizing them to identify areas where you find it challenging to monitor your expenditure.

5.    **<u>Don't commit to any new monthly bills:</u>** it just doesn't mean you're supposed to take your revenue and credit for a particular loan. Many believe that the bank would not accept a credit card or a loan the bank cannot afford. Your bank is not aware of any other obligations that might prevent your payments on time, but

only your income and debt obligations in your credit report. Depending on your income or other month-to-month commitments, it depends on you to choose whether a regular monthly repayment comes.

6.  **Make sure you pay the best price:** you can make the best of your money comparison shopping and make sure you pay for products and services at the lowest prices. Search for discounts, coupons, and cheaper options whenever possible.

7.  **Save up for big purchases:** you will be better helped with money if the ability to delay gratification goes along. You will evaluate the need and even more time to compare costs if you postpone big purchases rather than sacrificing more essentials or adding your purchase to the credit card. By saving up instead of using credit when you pay interest on purchasing. 6 And if you save, rather than over bills or bonds, well, you don't have to deal with

the various consequences of missing such statements.

8. **<u>Credit cards are a terrible opponent of a spending enemy;</u>** they limit your credit card purchases. You turn to your credit cards if you're running out of cash without thinking about whether you can afford to pay the balance. Resist the urge to use your credit cards, especially items you don't need for your purchases.

9. **<u>Regular contributions to savings:</u>** Every month, money can help you develop healthy financial habits in a savings account. You can also establish it as much as transfer money from your bank account to your savings account automatically. You need not remember to make the transfer in this way8.

10. **<u>Good with money Takes practice:</u>** You can't plan and delay buys until you can afford them initially. The more comfortable you make these habits part of your everyday life, the better

your money is handled, and your finances are better off.

Did you ever think, "Why are rich and poor remain poor? 'The answer, well, it's money-making. Getting money isn't going to make you rich. No matter how much you earn, it's like filling a bottle with a hole. If you don't use it lawfully, it will not be full no matter how much you fill. Money is an essential component of our life. We make a living and live. **In return, you can give your money a prosperous future through some calculated ways of spending. Here are five easy ways to preserve your wealth:**

a)      Earnings may come and go, but savings will be available during difficult times. Save a minimum of 10% of your monthly revenue. You shouldn't consider it to be the return for that specific month if you benefit from your business or compensation. In the past few months or years since you began your business or started working, it will be your return to work. The profit you earn over a month also illustrates how much you can make in the future. Do you agree? Do you agree? If so, you keep a reserve for the future of at least 10% (the more, the better).

b)   <u>Your savings investment:</u> your money's going to multiply. Twice is better all the time. Money that has remained idle or is not used is not saved as money. You will restrict yourself from growth if your savings are not invested or utilized. The more you spare and contribute today, the better you can spend later on. You are investing in a profitable venture.

c)    Tell your debt a Solid NO: You rob your future self every time you take a loan. The debt has eaten your financial income and also your next earnings. Often debts can keep you from growing. And whatever restricts your growth should be avoided. Usually, due to spending patterns, debts are taken. Avoid unnecessary small costs that help you spend on your income.

d)    Make your investment wisely: only make long-term benefits from calculated investments. You saw a disclaimer at the end of every investment ad: investments face market risks and the like? It is shown in the ads because it is necessary to choose investments in all the advantages and disadvantages. BEWARE: Know all risk, return, and informed decisions before investing. If necessary, consult experts.

Yes, you are your company's greatest asset. Learn new skills, polish, and use your current skills. It's part of our everyday lives to talk to people. Why not help? Why not?

✓ Everybody you meet must be **OBSERVE**

✓ **LEARN** from all the people you meet; every person will be teaching you something.

✓ Good study **IMPLEMENT**

✓ It will grow to be the most refined version of yourself, and you will be unresolvable.

1. How can I inculcate the habit of managing my resources?

2. What are the ways of maintaining my resources?

3. How do I deal with my money?

4. Why should I observe everyone I met?

**Note yourself Improvement in this chapter**

_____

_____

_____

_____

_____

_____

_____

_____

_____

_____

_____

_____

_____

_____

_____

-------------------------------------------------------

-------------------------------------------------------

-------------------------------------------------------

-------------------------------------------------------

-------------------------------------------------------

## TIPS FOR TAKING COMPLETE CONTROL OF YOUR LIFE

Life is made up of 10% of what happens to you and 90% of how you respond to it. Swindoll, Charles R.

Most of us go through life feeling as though we have no control over our lives.

Our time is consumed by tasks that must be completed, while our dreams are consumed by tasks that we believe we cannot complete. The majority of our conduct is dictated by social and financial commitments, while the remainder of our choices are limited by fear.

Life devolves into a sequence of events that occur to us.

But this does not have to be the case. You will overcome the anxieties and remove the external impediments that are keeping you back step by step. You can reclaim power. Your life has the potential to be yours. It is how it is done.

✓ **At least once a week, do something that scares you.**

Far too often, anxiety prevents us from accomplishing our goals in life. When you make it a habit to face your fears, you become numb to them. Then you begin to break free from the arbitrary self-imposed limitations that fear imposes.

- **Related reading:** Embracing the suck and developing mental toughness.

✓ **Sleep daily**

Sleep for 7–8 hours a night. Every day, go to bed and wake up about the same time. The precise time is unimportant; you could sleep from 10–5, 12–8, or even 3–10. What matters is that you keep a daily schedule so that your brain can maintain a healthy circadian rhythm. This consistency, in turn, makes it easier to structure and organize your life.

In terms of treatment, I don't want to give the impression that you can buy your way out of this issue, but I've noticed that low-dose (.5–1.5 mg) melatonin, combined with magnesium threonate, has helped many of my clients. Furthermore, using the Philips Go-Lite to expose your eyes to blue light during the day seems to help improve the day/night comparison, allowing you to be more alert during the day and sleepier at night.

It is an incredibly important subject, and you should certainly learn more about it. Begin with the three articles mentioned below: ten lifestyle changes that alleviated my onset insomnia, How to Sleep Well and Generate More Testosterone Every Night, as well as The Full Guide to Insomnia Cure

✓ **Save your funds**

A few wonderful things occur when you have some spare money saved up. You can afford to spoil yourself now and then without worrying about the cost. A significant portion of your life's burden is relieved. Perhaps most importantly, when you live within your means, you no longer have to make life decisions to increase your income; instead, you can prioritize other items, such as work-life balance or pursuing your passions.

However, don't try to save money by preceding a regular cup of coffee or, god forbid, avocado toast. Setting up a savings account and setting up an automatic transfer from your checking account to that savings account every payday is the simplest and most convenient way to save money. When you don't see the money initially, you won't even know it's gone.

✓   **Limit the use of caffeine and alcohol.**

Both have their uses: alcohol for relaxing and socializing and caffeine for staying awake in the mornings. However, the majority of people who eat them do so in excess. Try cutting your intake in half; you'll most likely get the same, if not more, benefits. Even better, you'll no longer be dependent on caffeine and alcohol to feel nice.

- **More reading:** How to Quit Caffeine Addiction in 4 Days Without Withdrawal Symptoms? A comprehensive guide to stopping coffee, as well as ten(10) caffeine alternatives you may not have considered.

✓ **Rent rather than buy**

Renting has several benefits over buying. You know what costs you per month, and you are not liable for any unexpected repair or maintenance costs. You will move with far less notice than a homeowner. You may also diversify your assets rather than buying a single asset worth 500% of your net worth.

- Bottom line: when you own a house, you often own a collection of responsibilities.

✓ **Reduce the time spent on social media.**

The most common way people waste time when they should be doing something else is via social media. Worse, it isn't often enjoyable- social media has devolved into a cesspool of needless debates, toxic social comparison, and detailed picture management.

Social networking is a useful tool for staying in contact with friends and organizing activities, but you shouldn't spend too much time on it. Check Facebook once a day and concentrate on your real life.

✓ **Create a side business**

Having a second income has the same advantages as saving money: less stress and greater financial independence. But it gets okay: There is no limit on how much money you can make with a side company, and you know that if you lose your job—or leave it—you can spend more time on your business and scale it up. It assists you with a great deal of versatility.

✓ **Maintain a tidy and organized home and workspace.**

Remove the actual clutter, and you remove the emotional clutter, allowing you to concentrate on what you're doing rather than how chaotic your surroundings are.

✓ **Expand the network**

Maintain contact with people in your business. Present in social events where you can meet new people. Don't think about what you'll get out of it right now; instead, focus on providing value to others. You'll need your network someday, and you must develop it before you need it.

✓ **Once a week, quick**

Once a week, fast for 24 hours without eating anything. It is a simple way to lose weight because it cuts the amount of time you eat per week 6/7. But, most importantly, learning not to succumb to hunger changes the relationship with food. Eating becomes a choice rather than something you have to do because you are hungry.

■ **Further reading:** Weight loss meal plans, diet schedule, and fasting

✓ **Put poverty into practice**

On this one, Let's take a look at Seneca quote:

Set aside a certain number of days to be comfortable with the scantiest and cheapest fare, with coarse and rough clothing, thus asking yourself, "Is this the situation that I feared?" It is precise during periods of immunity from treatment that the soul should toughen itself in preparation for times of greater stress. It is precisely during times of Fortune's kindness that it should fortify itself against her abuse. In times of calm, the soldier conducts maneuvers, builds earthworks with no enemy in sight, and exhausts himself with unnecessary toil to be ready for inevitable toil. If you don't want a man to flinch when a crisis strikes, prepare him before it happens.

### ✓ Trim any fat or bulk up a little.

Most people will benefit from this in terms of their well-being. But, even though you're already at a good weight, there's another significant psychological incentive to gain or lose weight: to prove to yourself that you can. If you've never consciously gained or lost weight before, doing so once will give you a tremendous sense of mastery over your own body.

- **More reading:** Roadmap to Ripped: A Comprehensive Step-by-Step Guide to Transforming Your Body from Obese to Shredded, or Anywhere in Between Also, I mentor people on this (along with sleep and building a healthy lifestyle).

✓ **Be ready for the worst.**

Determine what you are most afraid of, such as losing your career, having your house burn down, or contracting a serious illness. Create clear plans to a) minimize the likelihood of any of those events and b) react if and when they occur.

When we are afraid of something uncertain or poorly described, we are most afraid. Once you've considered how you'd cope with the thing you're afraid of, it would significantly reduce the anxiety you're experiencing.

✓ **Create a short to-do list for each day.**

The maximum of three products, and a minimum of the better; Many of the world's most productive people only assign themselves one major task every day. Concentrate on what is most important and fail to load your calendar with unnecessary tasks.

✓ **Eliminate things from your life.**

Objects that are no longer in use should be discarded. Stop engaging in things that aren't adding value to your life. Stop spending time with people whose business you dislike. Make space in your life for the important things to you, not only time but also physical and emotional resources.

✓ **Refuse almost anything.**

For the same purpose that you should eliminate things from your life, you should also avoid the temptation to add things that would consume your time and energy. Understand that something you add to your life has the power to dispense with other things you might be doing with your time and resources. Before taking on a new responsibility, ask yourself, "Does this deserve to be in my life?" The majority of the time, the answer would be no.

✓     **Modify your wardrobe**

One of the best pieces of advice I ever got came from the director of my college major program. She advised my class to always dress professionally for interviews, even though they were over the internet. Your clothing is an external manifestation of your self-image. When you change your clothing, you change your behavior and even your perception of yourself. Dress as if you are the person you want to be.

✓     **Make new friends.**

Meet new people who share some of your interests, particularly those you don't share with your current friends. Can accomplish this by searching for events on local news websites, Facebook, or Meetup.com.

Many people believe that they can't do things that their peers aren't interested in or have to do things because someone else is. Your social network becomes a source of liberation rather than restraint until you realize you have the opportunity to make new friends.

Aside from that, your social life has a major impact on your fitness. On the one hand, maintaining an active social life is beneficial to your well-being. Unhealthy friends and family, on the other hand, can influence you to be unhealthy. You must be prepared to deal with them to avoid or disarm social pressure; better yet, surround yourself with positive influences.

✓     **Take a ride by yourself.**

Please choose a region of the planet, or even a region of your own country, and spend at least a week exploring it yourself. It is not only enjoyable, but it also fosters independence, which will carry over into the rest of your life.

✓ **Consider it to be a decision.**

Stop telling yourself that you can't do anything unless it's physically impossible. Instead, tell you won't, because you have other interests or that you're unable to put in the effort.

Reflexively saying can't all the time teaches us to ignore every potential course of action that isn't obvious and easy. By quenching the word from your vocabulary, you would prepare yourself to seriously consider whether anything is possible rather than dismissing it as unlikely.

# CONCLUSION

At some point, the majority of us have said to ourselves, "I need to take better care of myself." Unfortunately, our dedication is often precipitated by sickness, exhaustion, or a life-altering occurrence in the worst-case scenario. We recognize the value of self-care but consistently place it on the back burner. Interestingly, even those who are not motivated to improve their health initially experience increased motivation once they begin. The secret to getting started is to begin. Once you begin, it's as if the rest of your system follows suit. Our organism is designed to maintain equilibrium.

Self-care entails much more than taking supplements and going to the gym. Our bodies are just a small part of our overall well-being. A healthy self-care regimen takes into account the mind, body, and soul.

Sometimes, our emotional and mental health has a profound effect on our physical health. Some of us take excellent care of our bodies but pay little attention to our emotions, stress levels, or negative self-talk regularly, all of which are just as harmful as the toxins found in our food and environment. Some of us (raising my hand sheepishly) take excellent care of our mental and emotional well-being by reading books, listening to inspirational audios, attending lectures, meditating, being with and expressing our feelings in healthy ways, but pay little attention to our bodies' signs and requests for assistance.

Printed in Great Britain
by Amazon